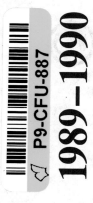

1989–1990

POCKETBOOK OF INFECTIOUS DISEASE THERAPY

John Bartlett, M.D.

Chief, Division of Infectious Diseases
The Johns Hopkins University School of Medicine
and The Johns Hopkins Hospital
Baltimore, Maryland

WILLIAMS & WILKINS

Baltimore • Hong Kong • London • Sydney

Editor: Timothy S. Satterfield
Associate Editor: Marjorie Kidd Keating
Copy Editor: Megan Westerfeld
Designer: Wilma Rosenberger
Illustration Planner: Lorraine Wrzosek
Production Coordinator: Raymond E. Reter

Copyright © 1990
Williams & Wilkins
428 East Preston Street
Baltimore, Maryland 21202, USA

Accurate indications, adverse reactions, and dosage schedules for drugs are provided in this book, but it is possible that they may change. The reader is urged to review the package information data of the manufacturers of the medications mentioned.

Printed in the United States of America

ISBN 0-683-00439-5

1 2 3 4 5 6 7 8 9 10

89 90 91 92 93

PREFACE

This book is intended for physicians and other care providers who manage adult patients with infectious diseases. This includes internists, generalists, surgeons, obstetricians and gynecologists. Its counterpart for pediatric care is the 1989-1990 Pocketbook of Pediatric Antimicrobial Therapy by Dr. John D. Nelson.

Many surveys in the 1970s indicated widespread misuse of antimicrobial agents. The glut of new antimicrobial agents and other evolutionary changes in the field of infectious diseases has made proper management even more difficult since that time. An obvious goal of this book is to provide acceptable standards for the care of patients with infections involving heterogeneous microbes at diverse anatomical sites.

There are many books that share in these goals. An obvious question concerns the need for yet another. Nearly any physician who has spent over 20 years practicing the discipline of infectious diseases believes he/she can provide a better therapeutic manual. Although this applies here as well, the most unique aspect of the book is the extensive use of guidelines from authoritative sources. Examples are the recommendations for managing tuberculosis by the American Thoracic Society, surgical prophylaxis according to consultants to The Medical Letter, treatment of sexually transmitted diseases by the Centers for Disease Control, treatment of endocarditis by the American Heart Association, recommendations for doses and dose adjustments for antimicrobial agents by the American Hospital Formulary Service and so forth. The author has inserted his own bias in selected areas where there are no guidelines from appropriate sources or where more recent data would modify prior recommendations.

The 1989-1990 Pocketbook of Infectious Disease Therapy will be revised annually with updated data and the addition of new topics. This is viewed as especially important in a field characterized by the constant influx of new drugs, periodic modifications of prior guidelines by the quoted authoritative sources and some conditions such as AIDS that are subject to rapid changes.

The author would like to thank Colleen Townsley for her tireless devotion to this work.

TABLE OF CONTENTS

PREPARATIONS AND RECOMMENDED DOSING REGIMENS FOR ANTIMICROBIAL AGENTS (ADAPTED FROM DRUG INFORMATION 88, AMERICAN HOSPITAL FORMULARY SERVICE, pp 31-463,1988)

Agent	Trade Names	Dosage Form	Usual Adult Regimen: Daily Dose, Route & Dose Interval
Acyclovir	Zovirax	5% ointment 200 mg caps 500 mg vials (IV)	Topical q3h 200-800 mg po; x 2-5/day 15-36 mg/kg/day IV over 1-3 hr q8h
Amantadine	Symmetrel	100 mg cap & tabs 50 mg/5 ml syrup	100-200 mg/day po q12-24h
Amdinocillin	Coactin	0.5; 1 gm vial	40-60 mg/kg/day IM or IV q4-6h
Amikacin	Amikin	0.1; 0.5; 1 gm vials	15 mg/kg/day IV q8-12h
Aminosalicylic acid	PAS	0.5 gm tab	150 mg/kg/day po q6-12h
Amoxicillin	Amoxil, Polymox, Trimox, Utimox, Wymox	250; 500 mg caps. 125; 250 mg/5 ml syrup	.75-2 gm/day po q6-8h
Amoxicillin + K clavulanate	Augmentin	125/31 mg/5 ml susp 250/62 mg/5 ml susp 250/125 mg tab 500/125 mg tab	.75-1.5 gm/day (amoxicillin) po q8h
Amphotericin B	Fungizone	50 mg vial	0.3-1 mg/kg/day IV over 4-8 hr q 1-2 days
Ampicillin	Omnipen, Amcill, Penamp, Polycillin, Principen, Totacillin	250;500 mg cap 125; 250; 500 mg/ 5 ml susp	1-2 gm/day po q6h
Ampicillin sodium	Omnipen-N, Polycillin-N, Totacillin-N	0.125; 0.25; 0.5; 1; 2; 10 gm vials	2-8 gm/day IV q4-6h
Ampicillin + sulbactam	Unasyn	1:0.5 gm + 2:1.0 gm vials (Ampsulbactam)	4-8 gm ampicillin/ day IV or IM q6h

(continued)

1

Agent	Trade Names	Dosage Form	Usual Adult Regimen: Daily Dose, Route & Dose Interval
Azlocillin	Azlin	2; 3; 4 gm vials	8-24 gm/day IV q 6-8 h
Aztreonam	Azactam	0.5; 1; 2 gm vials	1.5-6 gm/day IV or IM q6-8h
Bacampicillin	Spectrobid	400 mg tabs (equivalent to 280 mg ampicillin) 125 mg/5 ml syrup (equiv to 87 mg amp)	.8-1.6 gm/day po q12h
Bacitracin		10,000; 50,000 unit vials	10,000-25,000 units IM q6h 25,000 units po q6h
Capreomycin	Capastat	1 gm vial	1 gm/day IM
Carbenicillin disodium	Geopen, Pyopen	1;2;5;10;30 gm vials	8-40 gm/day IV q4-6h
Carbenicillin indanyl sodium	Geocillin	382 mg tabs	382-764 mg po q6h
Cefaclor	Ceclor	250;500 mg caps 125, 250 mg/5 ml syrup	1-2 gm/day po q6h
Cefadroxil	Duricef, Ultracef	500 mg caps; 1 gm tab; 125; 250; 500 mg/5 ml susp	1-2 gm/day po 1-2 x/day
Cefamandole nafate	Mandol	0.5;1;2;10 gm vials	2-18 gm/day IM or IV q4-6h
Cefazolin	Ancef, Kefzol	0.25;0.5; 1;5;10 gm vials	2-6 gm/day IV or IM q8h
Cefonicid	Monocid	0.5;1;2;6 gm vials	1-2 gm/day IV or IM in 1 dose/day
Cefoperazone	Cefobid	1;2 gm vials	2-8 gm/day IM or IV q8-12h
Ceforanide lysine	Precef	0.5;1;10 gm vials	1-3 gm/day IV or IM q12h

2

(continued)

Agent	Trade Names	Dosage Form	Usual Adult Regimen: Daily Dose, Route & Dose Interval
Cefotaxime sodium	Claforan	1;2;10 gm vials	2-12 gm/day IV or IM q6h
Cefotetan	Cefotan	1;2 gm vials	2-4 gm/day IV or IM q12h
Cefoxitin sodium	Mefoxin	1;2;10 gm vials	2-18 gm/day IV or IM q4-6h
Ceftazidime	Fortaz, Tazidime, Tazicef	0.5;1;2;6 gm vials	3-6 gm/day IV or IM q8-12h
Ceftizoxime sodium	Cefizox	1;2;10 gm vials	2-12 gm/day IV or IM q6-8h
Ceftriaxone	Rocephin	0.25;5;1;2;10 gm vial	1-4 gm IV or IM 1-2 doses/day
Cefuroxime	Zinacef	0.75;1.5 gm vial	2.25-4.5 gm/day IV or IM q6-8h
Cefuroxime axetil	Ceftin	0.125;0.25 gm cap	0.5-1.0 gm/day po q12h
Cephalexin monohydrate	Keflex	0.25;0.5;1 gm cap 125;250 mg/5 ml susp	1-2 gm/day po q6h
Cephalothin sodium	Keflin	1;2;4;10 gm vials	2-12 gm/day IV q4-6h
Cephapirin sodium	Cefadyl	1;2;4 gm vials	2-4 gm/day q6h
Cephradine	Anspor	250; 500 mg caps 125; 250 mg/5 ml susp	1-2 gm/day po q6h
	Velosef	0.25;0.5;1 gm vials	2-8 gm/day IV or IM q6h
Chloramphenicol	Chloromycetin	250 mg cap	1-2 gm/day po q6h
Chloramphenicol palmitate	Chloromycetin palmitate	150 mg/5 ml syrup	1-2 gm/day po q6h

(continued)

3

Agent	Trade Names	Dosage Form	Usual Adult Regimen: Daily Dose, Route & Dose Interval
Chloramphenicol Na succinate	Chloromycetin sodium succinate	1 gm vial	2-4 gm/day IV q6h
Chloroquine HCl	Aralen HCl	250 mg amp (200 mg base)	5 mg base/kg IM
Chloroquine PO4	Aralen PO4	500 mg tab (300 mg base) 250 mg tab (150 mg base)	300-600 mg (base) qd - q week
Chloroquine hydroxy	Plaquenil	200 mg tab (155 mg base)	10 mg/kg/day po q24h
Cinoxacin	Cinobac	250;500 mg cap	1 gm/day po q6-12h
Ciprofloxacin	Cipro	250;500;750 mg tabs	0.5-1.5 gm/day po q12h
Clindamycin HCl	Cleocin	75;150 mg cap	0.6-1.8 gm/day po q6-8h
Clindamycin PO4	Cleocin	150 mg/ml in vials (2,4,6 ml)	1.8-2.7 gm/day IV q6-8h
Clindamycin palmitate HCl	Cleocin pediatric	75 mg/5 ml solution	0.6-1.8 gm/day po q6-8h
Clofazimine	Lamprene	50;100 mg caps	50-300 mg/day po q8-24h
Cloxacillin Na	Tegopen Cloxapen	250; 500 mg cap 125 mg/5 ml solution	1-2 gm/day po q6h
Colistimethate Na	Coly-Mycin	150 mg (IM or IV) vial	2.5-5.0 mg/kg IV or IM q6-12h
Colistin S04	Coly-Mycin S	25 mg/5 ml susp 150 mg vial (IV)	2.5-5.0 mg/kg/day q6-12h
Cyclacillin	Cyclapen-W	250; 500 mg cap 125; 250 mg/5 ml susp	1-2 gm/day po q6h
Cycloserine	Seromycin	250 mg cap	0.5-1 gm/day po in 2 doses **(continued)**

4

Agent	Trade Names	Dosage Form	Usual Adult Regimen: Daily Dose, Route & Dose Interval
Dapsone		25, 100 mg tab	1-2 mg/kg/day po q24h
DHPG	Ganciclovir	500 mg vial	Initial: 10 mg/kg/day q12h; Maintenance: 5-6 mg/kg/day
Demeclocycline	Declomycin	125 mg cap 150; 300 mg cap	600 mg/day po q6-12h
Dicloxacillin	Dycill, Dynapen Pathocil	125; 250; 500 mg cap 62.5 mg/5 ml susp	1-2 gm/day po q6h
Doxycycline	Vibramycin Doxy caps Doxychel etc.	50 mg/5 ml susp 100 mg tabs 50;100 mg caps 100,200 mg vial	100-200 mg/day po q12-24h

200 mg/day IV q12h |
Emetine HCl		65 mg/ml	1 mg/kg/day up to 65 mg/day; IM or deep SC injection
Erythromycin base	E-mycin; ERYC; Ery-Tab Erythromycin Base Ilotycin, Pediamycin, Robimycin	125;250 mg caps 250;333;500 mg tabs 2% topical	1-2 gm/day po q6h (topical for acne)
Erythromycin estolate	Ilosone	250 mg caps, 125;250;500 mg tabs 125;250;500 mg/ 5 ml susp	1-2 gm/day po q6h
Erythromycin ethylsuccinate	E.E.S.; E-Mycin Ery Ped, Pediamycin, Wyamycin	200;400 mg tabs 100;200;400 mg/ 5 ml susp	1.6-3.2 gm/day po q6h
Erythromycin gluceptate	Ilotycin gluceptate	0.25; 0.5; 1 gm vial	2-4 gm/day IV q6h
Erythromycin lactobionate	Erythrocin lactobionate	0.5; 1 gm vial	1-4 gm/day IV q6h

(continued)

5

Agent	Trade Names	Dosage Form	Usual Adult Regimen: Daily Dose, Route & Dose Interval
Erythromycin stearate	Eramycin, Erypar; Erythrocin stearate; Ethril, Wyamycin S SK-erythromycin	250;500 mg tab	1-2 gm/day po q6h
Ethambutol hydrochloride	Myambutal	400 mg tab	15 mg/kg/day po q24h
Ethionamide	Trecator-SC	250 mg tab	0.5-1 gm/day po in 1-3 daily doses
Flucytosine	Ancobon	250; 500 mg cap	50-150 mg/kg/day po q6h
Furazolidone	Furoxone	100 mg tab	100 mg po q6h
Gentamicin SO4	Garamycin, Gentamicin SO4 Injection Isotonic (NaCl), Gentamicin SO4 ADD-Vantage, Gentamicin SO4 in 5% dextrose piggyback	0.4-2.4 mg/ml in 40-120 mg vials, 10 mg & 40 mg/ml, 60,80 & 100 mg vials, 2 mg/ml for intrathecal use	3-5 mg/kg/day IV or IM q8h
Griseofulvin	Grisactin, Fulvicin U/F, Grifulvin V, Gris-PEG, Grisactin Ultra, Fulvicin P/G	microsize: 125; 250; caps, 250;500 mg tab, 125 mg/5 ml susp ultramicrosize: 125; 165;250;330 mg tab	500 mg - 1 gm po/day
Imipenem/ Cilastatin	Primaxin	0.25;0.5 gm vials	1-4 gm/day IV q6h
Iodoquinol	Yodoxin	210 mg tab, 650 mg tab	650 mg/day po q8h
Isoniazid	Laniazid	50,100;300 mg tab, 50 mg/5 ml (oral solu), 1 gm vial (IM)	300 mg/day po q24h, 300 mg/day IM q12-24h (continued)

Agent	Trade Names	Dosage Form	Usual Adult Regimen: Daily Dose, Route & Dose Interval
Kanamycin SO4	Kantrex Klebcil	.075;0.5;1 gm vial 500 mg caps	15 mg/kg/day IV q8h
Ketoconazole	Nizoral	200 mg tab	200-400 mg/day po q 12-24 hr up to 1.6 gm/day
Mebendazole	Vermox	100 mg tab	100 mg po x 1-2 up to 2 gm/day
Methenamine hippurate	Hiprex	1 gm tabs	1-2 gm/day po q12h
Methenamine mandelate	Mandelamine	0.35;0.5;1 gm tab 250;500 mg/5 ml syrup 0.5;1 gm granules	1-4 gm/day po q6h
Methicillin Na	Celbenin Staphcillin	1;4;6;10 gm vial	4-12 gm/day IV or IM q6h
Metronidazole	Flagyl, Metryl Metizol, Protostat Metric 21, Satric	250;500 mg tab 500 mg vial	0.75-2 gm/day po q12h 0.75-2 gm/day IV q6-12h
Mezlocillin Na	Mezlin	1;2;3;4 gm vial	6-24 gm/day IV q4-6h
Miconazole	Monistat	200 mg amp	0.6-3.6 gm/day IV q8h
Minocycline HCl	Minocin	50;100 mg cap 50 mg/5 ml syrup 100 mg vial	200 mg/day po q12h 200 mg/day IV q12h
Moxalactam	Moxam	1;2;10 gm vial	2-8 gm/day IV q6-8h
Nafcillin Na	Unipen	250 mg caps; 500 mg tabs 250 mg/5 ml solu 0.5;1;2 gm vial	1-2 gm/day po q6h
	Nafcil, Nallpen, Unipen		2-12 gm/day IV or IM q4-6h
Nalidixic acid	NegGram	0.25; 0.5; 1 gm tab 250 mg/5 ml susp	1 gm po q6h

7

(continued)

Agent	Trade Names	Dosage Form	Usual Adult Regimen: Daily Dose, Route & Dose Interval
Neomycin SO4	Mycifradin	500 mg tab 125 mg/5 ml solu 500 mg vial for IM	3-12 gm po/day
Netilmicin	Netromycin	50; 150 mg vial	4-6.5 mg/kg/day IV or IM q8h
Niclosamide	Niclocide	500 mg tabs	2 gm (single dose)
Nitrofurantoin	Macrodantin Furantoin Furaton Furalan Faran	macrocrystals: 25; 50; 100 mg caps microcrystals: 50; 100 caps/tabs 25 mg/5 ml susp	50-100 mg po q6h
Norfloxacin	Noroxin	400 mg tabs	400 mg po bid
Novobiocin	Albamycin	250 mg caps	1-2 gm/day po q6-12h
Paromomycin SO4	Humatin	250 mg caps	3-4 gm/day po in 2-4 doses
Nystatin	Mycostatin Nystex Nilstat	100,000 units/ml susp 500,000 units tab	0.5 ml-1 mil units po 3-5 x daily
Oxacillin	Bactocill Prostaphlin	250; 500 mg caps 250 mg/5 ml solu 0.25; 0.5; 1; 2; 4; 10 gm vials	2-4 gm/day po q6h 2-12 gm/day IV or IM q4-6h
Penicillin Crystalline G potassium	Pentids	0.2; 0.25; 0.4; 0.5; 0.8 million unit tabs 0.2; 0.25; 0.4 million units/5 ml	1-2 gm po/day q6h
Crystalline G potassium	Penicillin G for injection	0.2; 0.5; 1; 5; 10; 20 million unit vials	2-20 million units IV q4-6h
Crystalline G sodium	Penicillin G sodium for injection	5 million unit vial	2-20 million units IV q4-6h **(continued)**

8

Agent	Trade Names	Dosage Form	Usual Adult Regimen: Daily Dose, Route & Dose Interval
Benzathine	Bicillin Bicillin L-A Permapen	200,000 unit tabs 300,000; 600,000 units/ml vial	Not recommended po 1.2–2.4 mil units IM
Benzathine + procaine	Bicillin C-R	Benzathine: procaine/ml 150,000:150,000 units (10 ml) 300,000:150,000 units (1,2,4 ml) 450,000:150,000 units (2 ml)	1.2–2.4 mil units IM
Procaine	Crysticillin Duracillin Pfizerpen Wycillin	300,000 units (10 ml) 500,000 units (12 ml) 600,000 units (1,2,4 ml syringe)	0.6–4.8 mil units/day IM q6–12h
Phenoxyethyl penicillin (V)	Beepen, Betapen Pen-Vee K,V-Cillin K, Veetids, Ledercillin Penapar VK	125;250;500 mg tabs 125;250 ml/5 ml susp	1–2 gm/day po q6h
Pentamidine	Pentam	300 mg vial	4 mg/kg IV qd
Piperacillin	Pipracil	2;3;4;40 gm vials	6–24 gm/day IV q4–6h
Polymyxin B	Aerosporin	500,000 unit vials 1 mg = 1,000 units	1.5–2.5 mg/kg/day IM or IV q4–6h
Praziquantel	Biltricide	600 mg tabs	20–75 mg/kg/day po in 3 doses
Primaquine		15 mg tabs	15 mg po qd
Pyrazinamide		500 mg tabs	15–30 mg/kg/day po in 6–8 doses
Pyrimethamine	Daraprim	25 mg tabs	25 mg po q wk or daily
Pyrimethamine + sulfadoxine	Fansidar	Sulfa-500 mg plus pyrimeth - 25 mg	1 tab/wk 3 tabs (1 dose)
Quinacrine HCl	Atabrine	100 mg	300–800 mg po/day **(continued)**

9

Agent	Trade Names	Dosage Form	Usual Adult Regimen: Daily Dose, Route & Dose Interval
Quinine SO4	Legatrin, Quine 200,300	130;200;300;325 mg caps, 260;325 mg tabs	325 mg bid, 650 mg q8h po
Quinine dihydrochloride		IV available from CDC	
Rifampin	Rifadin	150;300 mg caps	600 mg/day po (TB), 600-1200 mg/day po (other indications)
Spectinomycin	Trobicin	2; 4 gm vials	2 gm IM x 1
Streptomycin		1 & 5 gm vial	1-2 gm IM/day
Sulfonamides Trisulfapyrimidines	Triple sulfa, Neotrizine	Sulfadiazine, Sulfamerazine & Sulfamethazine, 167 mg (each) tabs and 167 mg (each) /5 ml susp	2-4 gm/day po q4-8h
Sulfadiazine	Microsulfon	0.5 gm tabs	2-4 gm/day po q4-8h
Sulfamethoxazole	Gantanol	0.5; 1 gm tabs	1 gm po q8-12h
Sulfapyridine		0.5 gm tabs	2 gm/day po q6h
Sulfasalazine	Azulfidine	0.5 gm tabs, 0.25 mg/5 ml susp	3-4 gm/day po q6h
Sulfisoxazole	Gantrisin	0.5 gm tabs	4-8 gm/day po q4-6h
Tetracyclines Demeclocycline	Dechlomycin	150 mg cap, 150; 300 mg tab	600 mg/day po q12h
Doxycycline	Vibramycin	50; 100 mg tabs, 50; 100 mg caps, 50 mg/5 ml susp, 100 mg vials	100-200 mg/day po q12-24h, 200 mg/day IV q 12-24h

(continued)

Agent	Trade Names	Dosage Form	Usual Adult Regimen: Daily Dose, Route & Dose Interval
Minocycline	Minocin	50; 100 mg caps 50; 100 mg tabs 100 mg vials	100 mg/day po or IV q6-12h
Oxytetracycline	Oxymycin; Terramycin, EP Mycin,	250 mg cap 500 mg vial (IV) 50;123 mg/ml with lidocaine (IM)	1-2 gm/day po q6h 0.5-1 gm/day IV q12h
Tetracycline	Achromycin; Brodspec, Cyclopar Robitet, Tetracap, Sumycin, etc.	100;250;500 mg caps 250;500 mg tabs 125 mg/5 ml susp 250; 500 mg vials (IV)	1-2 gm/day po q6h 0.5-1 gm/day IV q12h (up to 4 gm/day)
Thiabendazole	Mintezol	500 mg tab 500 mg/5 ml susp	1-3 gm po/day
Ticarcillin	Ticar	1;3;6;20;30 gm vials	4-24 gm/day IV q4-6h
Ticarcillin + clavulanic acid	Timentin	3 gm ticarcillin + 100 mg CA vials	3 gm (ticarcillin) IV q4-6h
Tobramycin	Nebcin	20;60;80 & 1,200 mg vials	3-5 mg/kg/day IV or IM q8h
Trimethoprim	Proloprim	100;200 mg tabs	200 mg/day po q12-24h
Trimethoprim- sulfamethoxazole	Bactrim, Septra Cotrim	Trimethoprim:sulfa 40 mg:200 mg/5 ml susp 80 mg:400 mg tabs 160 mg:800 mg DS tabs 16 mg:80 mg/ml (IV)	2-20 mg/kg/day (trimethoprim) po or IV q6-8h
Vancomycin	Vancocin pulvules Vancocin HCl Vancocin HCl IV Lyphocin	125;250 mg caps 1;10 gm vials (solu) 0.5;1 gm vials (IV)	0.5-2 gm/day po q6h 1-2 gm/day IV q6-12h
Vidarabine	Vira-A	200 mg/ml	15 mg/kg/day IV
Zidovudine	Retrovir, AZT	100 mg caps	100-200 mg po q4h

11

Organism	Usual Disease	Preferred Agent	Alternatives
Achromobacter xylosoxidans	Meningitis, septicemia	Antipseudomonad penicillin (2)	Sulfa-trimethoprim
Acinetobacter calcoaceticus var antitratum (Herellea vaginicola); var lwoffi (Mima polymorpha)	Sepsis (esp line sepsis) Pneumonia Endocarditis Meningitis	Imipenem Sulfa-trimethoprim	Aminoglycoside (1) ± antipseudomonad penicillin Ciprofloxacin Cephalosporin - 3rd gen. (5) Sulfonamide
Actinobacillus acetomycetem-comitans	Actinomycosis Endocarditis	Penicillin	Clindamycin Tetracycline (4) Erythromycin Cephalosporins
Actinomyces israelii (also A. naeslundii, A. viscosus, A. odontolyticus and Arachnia proprionica)	Actinomycosis	Penicillin G	Clindamycin Tetracycline (4) Erythromycin
Aeromonas hydrophila	Diarrhea Bacteremia Cutaneous infections Meningitis	Sulfa-trimethoprim	Chloramphenicol Ciprofloxacin Aminoglycoside (1) Tetracycline (4) Imipenem Aztreonam Amoxicillin/Ticarcillin + clavulanic acid **(continued)**

12

Organism	Usual Disease	Preferred Agent	Alternatives
Bacillus anthracis	Anthrax	Penicillin G	Erythromycin Tetracycline (4) Chloramphenicol
Bacillus cereus	Food poisoning	Not treated	
Bacillus species	Septicemia (comp host)	Vancomycin	Imipenem Aminoglycosides (1)
Bacteroides bivius	Female genital tract infections	Metronidazole Clindamycin Cefoxitin	Cefotetan Chloramphenicol Antipseudomonad penicillin (2) Imipenem Ticarcillin-clavulanic acid Ampicillin-sulbactam
"B. fragilis group"	Abscesses Bacteremia Intra-abdominal sepsis	Metronidazole Clindamycin Cefoxitin Imipenem Ticarcillin-clavulanic acid	Cefotetan Chloramphenicol Antipseudomonad penicillin (2) Ampicillin-sulbactam
"B. melaninogenicus group"	Oral-dental & pulmonary infections Female genital tract infections	Metronidazole Clindamycin Cefoxitin	Chloramphenicol Penicillin G Ampicillin Imipenem Cefotetan
Bordetella pertussis	Pertussis	Erythromycin	Sulfa-trimethoprim (3)

(continued)

13

Organism	Usual Disease	Preferred Agent	Alternatives
Borrelia burgdorferi	Lyme disease	Tetracycline (early disease) Ceftriaxone (late complications)	Penicillin G po or IV Amoxicillin Erythromycin
Borrelia recurrentis	Relapsing fever	Tetracycline (4)	Penicillin G Erythromycin Chloramphenicol
Branhamella catarrhalis (Moraxella catarrhalis)	Otitis, sinusitis, pneumonitis	Sulfa-trimethoprim	Amoxicillin-clavulanic acid Erythromycin Tetracycline (4) Cefaclor Cephalosporin (3rd gen) (5) Cefuroxime
Brucella	Brucellosis	Tetracycline (4) + streptomycin or rifampin	Chloramphenicol + streptomycin Sulfa-trimethoprim
Calymmatibacterium granulomatis	Granuloma inguinale	Tetracycline (4)	Sulfa-trimethoprim Erythromycin (pregnancy) Gentamicin Chloramphenicol
Campylobacter jejuni	Diarrhea	Erythromycin	Tetracycline (4) Gentamicin Ciprofloxacin Chloramphenicol
Campylobacter fetus	Septicemia, vascular infections, meningitis	Gentamicin	Chloramphenicol

14

(continued)

Organism	Usual Disease	Preferred Agent	Alternatives
Capnocytophaga ochraceae	Periodontal disease Bacteremia in neutropenic host Tonsillitis (?)	Penicillins Clindamycin Erythromycin	Amoxicillin-clavulanic acid Imipenem Cefoxitin Cephalosporins (3rd gen) (5) Ciprofloxacin Tetracycline
Chlamydia psittaci	Psittacosis	Tetracycline (4)	Chloramphenicol
Chlamydia pneumoniae (TWAR agent)	Pneumonia	Tetracycline (4)	Erythromycin
Chlamydia trachomatis	Urethritis Endocervicitis PID Epididymitis Urethral syndrome	Tetracycline (4)	Ciprofloxacin Erythromycin
	Trachoma	Tetracycline (4) (topical + oral)	Sulfonamide (topical + oral)
	Lymphogranuloma venereum	Tetracycline (4)	Erythromycin
	Inclusion conjunctivitis	Erythromycin (topical or oral)	Sulfonamide
Citrobacter diversus	Urinary tract infections, Pneumonia	Aminoglycoside (1) Cephalosporin (2nd & 3rd generation) (5) Sulfa-trimethoprim	Tetracycline (4) Imipenem Ciprofloxacin/Norfloxacin

15

(continued)

Organism	Usual Disease	Preferred Agent	Alternatives
Citrobacter freundii	Urinary tract infection, wound infection, septicemia, pneumonia	Imipenem Sulfa-trimethoprim Aminoglycoside (Amikacin) Ciprofloxacin/Norfloxacin	Tetracycline (4) Cephalosporin (3rd generation) (5)
Clostridium difficile	Antibiotic-associated colitis	Vancomycin (oral) Metronidazole (oral)	Bacitracin (oral) Cholestyramine Lactobacilli
Clostridium sp.	Gas gangrene Sepsis Tetanus Botulism Crepitant cellulitis	Penicillin G	Chloramphenicol Metronidazole Erythromycin Antipseudomonad penicillin (2) Clindamycin
Corynebacterium diphtheriae	Diptheria	Erythromycin + antitoxin	Penicillin G
Corynebacterium JK strain	Septicemia	Vancomycin	Ciprofloxacin
Coxiella burnetii	Q fever	Tetracycline (4)	Chloramphenicol
DF-2	Septicemia (dog bite) Wound infection	Penicillin	Erythromycin
Edwardsiella tarda	Gastroenteritis Wound infection Bacteremia, liver abscesses	Ampicillin	Tetracycline (4) Cephalosporin (5) Aminoglycoside (1) Chloramphenicol **(continued)**

Organism	Usual Disease	Preferred Agent	Alternatives
Ehrlichia	Ehrlichiosis	Tetracycline (4)	
Eikenella corrodens	Oral infections, bite wounds	Ampicillin/amoxicillin Penicillin G	Tetracycline (4) Erythromycin Amoxicillin-clavulanic acid Cephalosporin (5)
Enterobacter aerogenes, E. cloacae	Sepsis, pneumonia, wound infection	Aminoglycoside (1) Cephalosporin - 3rd gen (5)	Aztreonam Imipenem Antipseudomonad penicillin (2) Sulfa-trimethoprim Ciprofloxacin
	Urinary tract infection infection	Sulfa-trimethoprim Cephalosporin - 3rd gen. (5)	Antipseudomonad penicillin (2) Aminoglycoside Ciprofloxacin/Norfloxacin Imipenem
Erwinia agglomerans	Urinary tract infection Bacteremia Pneumonia	Aminoglycoside (1)	Ciprofloxacin Chloramphenicol Cephalosporins
Erysipelothrix insidiosa	Sepsis, cellulitis, abscesses	Ampicillin + aminoglycoside (1)	Tetracycline (4)
E. coli	Septicemia Intra-abdominal sepsis Wound infection	Aminoglycoside (1) Cephalosporin (5)	Ampicillin Sulfa-trimethoprim Antipseudomonad penicillin (2) Imipenem Aztreonam **(continued)**

Organism	Usual Disease	Preferred Agent	Alternatives
	Urinary tract infection	Ampicillin Tetracycline (4) Sulfa-trimethoprim (3) Aminoglycoside (1) Cephalosporin (5) Antipseudomonad penicillin (2)	Imipenem Aztreonam Ciprofloxacin/Norfloxacin Sulfonamide
Flavobacterium meningosepticum	Sepsis	Vancomycin	Sulfa-trimethoprim
Francisella tularensis	Tularemia	Streptomycin or gentamicin	Tetracycline (4) Chloramphenicol
Fusobacterium	Oral/dental/pulmonary infection; liver abscess	Penicillin G	Cefoxitin/cefotetan Chloramphenicol Imipenem Clindamycin Metronidazole
Gardnerella vaginalis	Vaginitis	Metronidazole	Ampicillin
Haemophilus aphrophilus	Sepsis, endocarditis	Penicillin G + aminoglycoside (1)	Cephalosporin - 3rd gen (5) + aminoglycoside (1)
H. ducreyi	Chancroid	Ceftriaxone	Sulfa-trimethoprim Erythromycin Amoxicillin + clavulanic acid Ciprofloxacin **(continued)**

18

Organism	Usual Disease	Preferred Agent	Alternatives
H. influenzae	Meningitis	Cephalosporin-cefuroxime, cefotaxime, ceftriaxone Chloramphenicol $\pm$ ampicillin Cefamandole/cefuroxime	
	Epiglottitis Pneumonia Arthritis Cellulitis	Cephalosporin - 3rd gen (5) Sulfa-trimethoprim	Chloramphenicol $\pm$ ampicillin Ampicillin/ticarcillin - clavulanic acid
	Otitis Sinusitis Bronchitis	Sulfa-trimethoprim (3) Ampicillin/amoxicillin Amoxicillin - clavulanic acid	Erythromycin - sulfonamide Cefaclor Tetracycline (4)
Hafnia alvei	Pneumonia, wound infection, urinary tract infection	Aminoglycoside (1)	Ciprofloxacin Chloramphenicol Antipseudomonad penicillin (2)
Klebsiella pneumoniae, K. oxytoca	Septicemia Pneumonia Intra-abdominal sepsis	Cephalosporin $\pm$ aminoglycoside (1)	Aminoglycoside (1) Sulfa-trimethoprim Pipericillin/mezlocillin Imipenem Ticarcillin - clavulanic acid Aztreonam Ampicillin-sulbactam Ciprofloxacin **(continued)**

Organism	Usual Disease	Preferred Agent	Alternatives
	Urinary tract infection	Sulfa-trimethoprim Cephalosporin (5) Tetracycline (4)	Aminoglycoside (1) Amoxicillin/ticarcillin - clavulanic acid Ciprofloxacin/norfloxacin Pipericillin/mezlocillin Imipenem
Legionella sp.	Legionnaires' disease	Erythromycin $\pm$ rifampin	Sulfa-trimethoprim + rifampin
Leptospira	Leptospirosis	Penicillin G	Tetracycline (4)
Leptotrichia buccalis	Orodental infections	Penicillin G	Tetracycline (4) Clindamycin
Listeria monocytogenes	Meningitis Septicemia	Ampicillin $\pm$ gentamicin	Sulfa-trimethoprim Erythromycin
Moraxella	Ocular infections Bacteremia	Aminoglycoside (1) Penicillins	Cephalosporin - 3rd gen (5) Imipenem Ciprofloxacin
Moraxella catarrhalis (See Branhamella catarrhalis)			
Morganella morganii	Bacteremia Urinary tract infection Pneumonia Wound infection	Aminoglycoside (Amikacin) Ciprofloxacin/norfloxacin	Imipenem Aztreonam Antipseudomonad penicillin (2) Ticarcillin - clavulanic acid Amoxicillin - clavulanic acid Tetracycline (4) **(continued)**

Organism	Usual Disease	Preferred Agent	Alternatives
Mycobacterium tuberculosis	Tuberculosis	INH + rifampin $\pm$ pyrazinamide	Streptomycin Cycloserine Ethambutal Ethionamide Kanamycin Capreomycin PAS
M. kansasii	Pulmonary infection	INH + rifampin + ethambutal	Streptomycin Ethionamide Cycloserine
M. avium-intracellulare	Pulmonary infection Disseminated infection	INH + rifampin + ethambutal $\pm$ streptomycin	Clofazimine Capreomycin Ethionamide Amikacin Imipenem Cycloserine Ansamicin Ciprofloxacin
M. fortuitum	Soft tissue and wound infections	Amikacin + doxycycline	Rifampin Erythromycin Sulfonamide Cefoxitin
M. marinum	Soft tissue infections	Minocycline	Sulfa-trimethoprim Rifampin Cycloserine **(continued)**

Organism	Usual Disease	Preferred Agent	Alternatives
M. leprae	Leprosy	Dapsone + rifampin $\pm$ clofazimine	Rifampin Ethionamide (Prothionamide) Cycloserine
Mycoplasma pneumoniae	Pneumonia	Erythromycin Tetracycline (4)	
Neisseria gonorrhoeae	Urethritis Salpingitis Cervicitis Arthritis-dermatitis	Ceftriaxone	Penicillin G + probenecid Ampicillin or amoxicillin + probenecid Cefotaxime Cefoxitin Spectinomycin Sulfa-trimethoprim
Penicillinase-producing strains	(Same)	Ceftriaxone	Sulfa-trimethoprim Spectinomycin
N. meningitidis	Meningitis Bacteremia Pericarditis Pneumonia	Penicillin G	Ampicillin Chloramphenicol Sulfa-trimethoprim Cephalosporin-cefotaxime, ceftizoxime, ceftriaxone cefuroxime
Nocardia asteroides	Nocardiosis: pulmonary infection, abscesses - skin, lung, brain	Sulfonamide	Sulfa-trimethoprim Minocycline Amikacin Cycloserine **(continued)**

Organism	Usual Disease	Preferred Agent	Alternatives
Pasteurella multocida	Animal bite wound	Penicillin G	Tetracycline (4) Erythromycin Amoxicillin-clavulanic acid Cephalosporins Ampicillin-sulbactam
Peptostreptococcus	Oral/dental/pulmonary infection; intra-abdominal sepsis gynecologic infection	Penicillin G	Clindamycin Metronidazole Cephalosporin (5) Chloramphenicol Erythromycin Vancomycin Imipenem
Plesiomonas shigelloides	Diarrhea	Sulfa-trimethoprim Tetracycline (4) Ciprofloxacin	Chloramphenicol Aminoglycoside (1)
Propionibacterium acnes	Acne	Tetracycline (4)	Clindamycin (topical)
Proteus mirabilis	Septicemia Urinary tract infection Intra-abdominal sepsis Wound infection	Ampicillin	Aminoglycosides (1) Cephalosporins (2nd & 3rd) (5) Sulfa-trimethoprim Antipseudomonad penicillin Aztreonam Imipenem Ciprofloxacin
Proteus vulgaris	Septicemia Urinary tract infection	Cephalosporin - 3rd gen (5) Aminoglycoside (1)	Sulfa-trimethoprim Antipseudomonad penicillin (2) Aztreonam **(continued)**

23

Organism	Usual Disease	Preferred Agent	Alternatives
			Imipenem Amoxicillin/ticarcillin + clavulanic acid Ciprofloxacin
Providencia rettgeri	Septicemia Urinary tract infection	Cephalosporin - 3rd gen (5) Aminoglycoside (1)	Antipseudomonad penicillin (2) Imipenem Aztreonam Sulfa-trimethoprim
Providencia stuartii	Septicemia Urinary tract infections	Aminoglycoside (1) Cephalosporin - 3rd gen (5)	Antipseudomonad penicillin (2) Sulfa-trimethoprim Imipenem Aztreonam Ciprofloxacin

Pseudomonas
aeruginosa
	Septicemia, pneumonia
	Intra-abdominal sepsis
		Aminoglycoside (tobramycin)
		± antipseudomonad
		penicillin (2)
			Aminoglycoside (1) ±
			  Cefoperazone,
			  Imipenem or
			  Ceftazidime
			Aztreonam
			Ciprofloxacin

	Urinary tract infections	Aminoglycoside (1) Antipseudomonad penicillin (2)	Imipenem Ceftazidime Cefoperazone Aztreonam Ciprofloxacin/norfloxacin
Ps. cepacia	Septicemia Pneumonia	Sulfa-trimethoprim	Chloramphenicol Ceftazidime

Organism	Usual Disease	Preferred Agent	Alternatives
Ps. mallei	Glanders	Streptomycin + tetracycline	Chloramphenicol + streptomycin
Ps. maltophilia	Septicemia Pneumonia	Sulfa-trimethoprim	Ticarcillin-clavulanic acid
Ps. pseudomallei	Melioidosis	Sulfa-trimethoprim	Tetracycline (4) $\pm$ chloramphenicol Chloramphenicol $\pm$ aminoglycoside (1) Sulfonamide
Rickettsia	Rocky Mountain spotted fever, Q fever, tick bite fever, murine typhus, scrub typhus, typhus, trench fever	Tetracycline (4) (> 8 yrs)	Chloramphenicol
Salmonella typhi	Typhoid fever	Chloramphenicol	Sulfa-trimethoprim Ampicillin/amoxicillin Ciprofloxacin Cefotaxime/cefoperazone/ ceftriaxone
Salmonella sp. (other)	Enteric fever Mycotic aneurysm	Ampicillin/amoxicillin Sulfa-trimethoprim	Chloramphenicol Ciprofloxacin Cefotaxime/cefoperazone/ ceftriaxone
Serratia marcescens	Septicemia Urinary tract infection Pneumonia	Cephalosporin (3rd gen) (5) Gentamicin or amikacin $\pm$ antipseudomonad penicillin or cephalosporin-3rd gen (5)	Cephalosporins (3rd gen) (5) Sulfa-trimethoprim Antipseudomonad penicillin (2) Imipenem Ciprofloxacin Aztreonam **(continued)**

Organism	Usual Disease	Preferred Agent	Alternatives
Shigella	Colitis	Sulfa-trimethoprim	Ampicillin Tetracycline (4) Ciprofloxacin/Nalidixic acid
Spirillum minus	Rat bite fever	Penicillin G	Tetracycline (4) Streptomycin
Staphylococcus aureus Methicillin sensitive	Septicemia Pneumonia Wound infection Abscesses	Penicillinase resistant penicillin (3) $\pm$ rifampin or gentamicin Cephalosporins (1st gen) (5) Cefuroxime/cefamandole	Erythromycin/clindamycin Vancomycin Amoxicillin - clavulanic acid Ticarcillin - clavulanic acid Imipenem Ciprofloxacin Ampicillin - sulbactam
Methicillin resistant		Vancomycin $\pm$ rifampin or gentamicin	Sulfa-trimethoprim Ciprofloxacin Imipenem
Staph saprophyticus	Urinary tract infections	Sulfa-trimethoprim Ampicillin/Amoxicillin	Cephalosporins Tetracycline (4) Ciprofloxacin/Norfloxacin

Staph epidermidis	Septicemia
	Infected prosthetic
	  devices
		Vancomycin	Sulfa-trimethoprim
			Penicillinase resistant
			  penicillin
			Cephalosporin (5)
			Ciprofloxacin
			Imipenem

Organism	Usual Disease	Preferred Agent	Alternatives
Streptococcus, Group A,B,C,G; bovis, milleri, pneumoniae, viridans, anaerobic	Pharyngitis Soft tissue Pneumonia Abscesses	Penicillin G	Cephalosporin (5) Clindamycin Vancomycin Erythromycin
	Endocarditis	Penicillin G $\pm$ streptomycin or gentamicin	Cephalosporin (5) Vancomycin
	Meningitis	Penicillin G	Chloramphenicol Cephalosporin - 3rd gen (5)
Strep group D enterococcus (Enterococcus faecalis and E. faecium)	Urinary tract infection	Ampicillin/amoxicillin	Penicillin + aminoglycoside (1) Vancomycin Nitrofurantoin Ciprofloxacin/norfloxacin
	Wound infection Intra-abdominal sepsis	Ampicillin/amoxicillin	Vancomycin Penicillin + aminoglycoside (1) Imipenem
	Endocarditis	Penicillin G/ampicillin + gentamicin or streptomycin	Vancomycin + gentamicin or streptomycin
Strep moniliformis	Rat bite fever Haverhill fever	Penicillin G	Tetracycline (4) Streptomycin
Treponema pallidum	Syphilis	Penicillin G	Tetracycline (4) Erythromycin
Treponema pertenue	Yaws	Penicillin G	Tetracycline (4) **(continued)**

Organism	Usual Disease	Preferred Agent	Alternatives
Ureaplasma urealyticum	Urethritis Endocervicitis PID (?)	Erythromycin	Tetracycline (4)
Vibrio cholerae	Cholera	Tetracycline (4)	Sulfa-trimethoprim
Vibrio parahaemolyticus	Enterocolitis	Tetracycline (4)	Ciprofloxacin Furazolidine
Vibrio vulnificus	Septicemia Wound infection	Tetracycline (4) + aminoglycoside (1)	Chloramphenicol Penicillin G
Yersinia enterocolitica	Enterocolitis Mesenteric adenitis Septicemia	Sulfa-trimethoprim Aminoglycoside (gentamicin)	Cephalosporin - 3rd gen (5) Ciprofloxacin Tetracycline (4)
Yersinia pestis	Plague	Streptomycin	Chloramphenicol Tetracycline (4)
Yersinia pseudotuberculosis	Mesenteric adenitis	Aminoglycoside (1) Ampicillin	Sulfa-trimethoprim Tetracycline (4)

1. Aminoglycosides = Gentamicin, tobramycin, amikacin, netilmicin
2. Antipseudomonad penicillin = Carbenicillin, ticarcillin, piperacillin, mezlocillin, azlocillin
3. Penicillinase resistant penicillins: Nafcillin, oxacillin, methicillin, cloxacillin, dicloxacillin
4. Tetracycline = Tetracycline, doxycycline, minocycline
5. Cephalosporins
    1st generation: Cefadroxil, cefazolin, cephalexin, cephalothin, cephapirin, cephradine
    2nd generation: Cefaclor, cefamandole, cefonicid, ceforanide, cefotetan, cefoxitin, cefuroxime
    3rd generation: Cefotaxime, ceftizoxime, ceftazidime, cefoperazone, ceftriaxone, moxalactam

ANTIMICROBIAL REGIMENS IN RENAL FAILURE

A. General Principles

1. The initial dose is not modified.

2. Adjustments in subsequent doses for renally excreted drugs may be accomplished by **a)** giving the usual maintenance dose at extended intervals, usually 3 half lives (extended interval method); **b)** giving reduced doses at the usual intervals (dose reduction method) or **c)** a combination of each.

3. Adjustments in dose are usually based on creatinine clearance that may be estimated as follows:

   a. Formula: Males: $\dfrac{\text{weight (kg)} \times (140-\text{age in yrs})}{72 \times \text{serum creatinine (mg/dl)}}$

   Females: above value x 0.85

   b. Nomogram (Kampmann J et al. Acta Med Scand 196:617,1974).

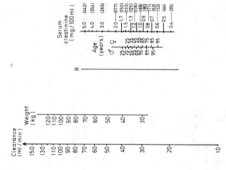

Use a straight edge to connect the patient's weight (2nd line on the left) and the patient's age (4th line). Mark intercept on R (3rd line) and swing straight edge to serum creatinine (5th line). Intercept on first line provides creatinine clearance.

c. Pitfalls and notations with calculations

(1) Elderly patient: Serum creatinine may be deceptively low (with danger of overdosing) due to reduced muscle mass.

(2) Pregnancy and volume expansion: GFR may be increased (with danger of underdosing) in third trimester of pregnancy and patients with normal renal function who receive massive parenteral fluids.

(3) Obese patients: Use lean body weight.

(4) Renal failure: Formulas assume stable renal function; for patients with anuria or oliguria assume CCr of 5-8 ml/min.

29

B. Aminoglycoside Dosing

1. Guidelines of Johns Hopkins Hospital Clinical Pharmacology Department

Agent	Loading dose (regardless of renal function)	Subsequent doses (prior to level measurements) CCr>70 ml/mm	CCr<70 ml/mm	Therapeutic levels (1 hr after infusion over 20-30 min)
Gentamicin	2 mg/kg	1.7-2 mg/kg/8h	.03 × CCr=mg/kg/8h	5-10 mcg/ml
Tobramycin	2 mg/kg	1.7-2 mg/kg/8h	.03 × CCr=mg/kg/8h	5-10 mg/ml
Netilmicin	2.2 mg/kg	2-2.2 mg/kg/8h	.03 × CCr=mg/kg/8h	5-10 mg/ml
Amikacin	8 mg/kg	7.5-8 mg/kg/8h	.12 × CCr=mg/kg/8h	20-40 mg/ml
Kanamycin	8 mg/kg	7.5-8 mg/kg/8h	.12 × CCr=mg/kg/8h	20-40 mg/ml

Note:
1. CCr = creatinine clearance.
2. Doses for gentamicin, tobramycin and netilmicin should be written in multiples of 5 mg; doses of amikacin and kanamycin should be written in multiples of 25 mg.
3. For obese patients use calculated lean body weight.
4. For patients who are oliguric or anuric use CCr of 5-8 ml/min.

2. Mayo Clinic guidelines (VanScoy RE and Wilson WR, Mayo Clin Proc 62:1142, 1987)
a. Initial dose: Gentamicin, tobramycin, netilmicin: 1.5-2 mg/kg
   Amikacin, kanamycin, streptomycin: 5.0-7.5 mg/kg
b. Maintenance dose: Usual daily dose × CCr/100

3. Reduced dose nomogram developed for tobramycin

Weight		Usual dose (q8h)	
lbs	kg	mg/kg	1.7 mg/kg
264	120	120	200
242	110	110	185
220	100	100	165
198	90	90	150
176	80	80	135
154	70	70	115
132	60	60	100
110	50	50	85
88	40	40	65

4. **Guidelines of AMA Drug Evaluations, 6th Edition, Chicago, 1986, p 1439 and Drug Information 88, American Hospital Formulary Service, 1988, p 58**

a. Loading dose based on estimated ideal body weight

Agent	Dose (mg/kg ideal wt)	Peak conc. (mcg/ml)
Tobramycin	1.5-2 mg/kg	4-10
Gentamicin	1.5-2 mg/kg	4-10
Netilmicin	1.3-3.25 mg/kg	4-12
Amikacin	5-7.5 mg/kg	15-30
Kanamycin	5-7.5 mg/kg	15-30

b. Maintenance dose as % of loading dose according to desired dosing interval and the corrected creatinine clearance CCr*

$$CCr\ (male) = \frac{(140 - age)}{serum\ creatinine}$$

$$CCr\ (female) = 0.85 \times CCr\ male$$

CCr (ml/min)	Half life (hrs)**	Dosing Interval (hr) 8	12	24
90	3.1	84%	-	-
80	3.4	80%	91%	-
70	3.9	76%	88%	-
60	4.5	71%	84%	-
50	5.3	65%	79%	-
40	6.5	57%	72%	92%
30	8.4	48%	63%	86%
25	9.9	43%	57%	81%
20	11.9	37%	50%	75%
17	13.6	33%	46%	70%
15	15.1	31%	42%	67%
12	17.9	27%	37%	61%
10***	20.4	24%	34%	56%
7	25.9	19%	28%	47%
5	31.5	16%	23%	41%
2	46.8	11%	16%	30%
0	69.3	8%	11%	21%

* From: Sarubbi FA JR, Hull JH. Ann Intern Med 89:612,1978.

** Maintenance dose may be one half the loading dose at an interval approximately the estimated half life.

*** Serum concentrations should be measured to assist dose selection when the CCr is < 10 ml/min.

Drug Therapy Dosing Guidelines
(Adapted from Bennett WM, et al: Ann Intern Med 93:62,1980 and AMA Drug Evaluations, 6th Ed, 1986, pp 1291-1631)

Drug	Major excretory route	Half life (hr) Normal	Half life (hr) Anuria	Usual regimen Oral	Usual regimen Parenteral	Maintenance regimen renal failure Glomerular filtration rate in mL/min 50-80	10-50	<10
Acyclovir	Renal	2-2.5	20	200-800 mg 2-5 x daily		Usual	200 mg 5x/day q12h	Usual q12h
					5-12 mg/kg q8h	Usual q8h	Usual q12-24h	50% of usual q24h
Amantidine	Renal	15-20	170	100 mg bid	-	100-150 mg q day	100-200 mg 2-3 x/wk	100-200 mg q wk
Amdinocillin	Renal	1.0	3.3	-	10 mg/kg q4-6h	Usual	10 mg/kg q6h	10 mg/kg q8h
Amikacin	Renal	2h	30h	-	7.5 mg/kg	See page 30,31		
Amoxicillin	Renal	1	15-20	250-500 mg q8h	-	.25-.5 gm q12h	.25-.5 gm q12-24h	.25-.5 gm q12-24h
Amoxicillin-clavulanic acid	Renal	1	8-16	250-500 mg q8h	-	Usual	0.25-0.5 gm q12h	0.25-0.5 gm q20-36h
Amphotericin B	Nonrenal	24	24	-	See pg 87,88	Usual	Usual	Usual
Ampicillin	Renal	1.0	8-12	.25-0.5 gm q6h	-	Usual	Usual	Usual
					1-3 gm q4-6h	Usual	1-2 gm IV q8h	1-2 gm IV q12h

(continued)

Drug	Major excretory route	Half life (hr) Normal	Half life (hr) Anuria	Usual regimen Oral	Usual regimen Parenteral	Maintenance regimen renal failure Glomerular filtration rate in mL/min 50-80	10-50	<10
Ampicillin-sulbactam	Renal	1.0	8-12h	-	1-2 gm q6h	102 gm IV q8h	1-2 gm IV q8h	1-2 gm IV q12h
Azlocillin	Renal	1	5	-	2-4 gm q4-6h	Usual	1.5-2gm q8h	1.5-3 gm q12h
Aztreonam	Renal	1.7-2	6-9	-	1-2 gm q6h	1-2 gm q8-12h	1-2 gm q12-18h	1-2 gm q24h
Bacampicillin	Renal			0.4-0.8 gm q12h	-	Usual	Usual	
Capreomycin	Renal	4-6	50-100	1 gm q day-2x/wk	-	Usual	7.5 mg/kg q 1-2 days	7.5 mg/kg 2 x/wk
Carbenicillin	Renal	1.0	13-16	.5-1 gm q6h -	- 5-6 gm IV q4h	Usual Usual	Usual 2-3 gm q6h	Avoid 2 gm q12h
Cefaclor	Renal	0.75	2.8	.25-0.5 gm q8h	-	Usual	Usual	Usual
Cefadroxil	Renal	1.4	20-25	.5-1 gm q12-24h	-	Usual	.5 gm q12-24h	.5 gm q36h
Cefamandole	Renal	0.5-1.0	10	-	0.5-2 gm q4-8h	.5-2 gm q6h	1-2 gm q8h	0.5-1 gm q12h
Cefazolin	Renal	1.8	18-36	-	0.5-2 gm q8h	0.5-1.5 gm q8h	.5-1 gm q8-12h	0.25-0.75 gm q18-24h

(continued)

33

Drug	Major excretory route	Half life (hr) Normal	Anuria	Usual regimen Oral	Parenteral	Maintenance regimen renal failure Glomerular filtration rate in mL/min 50-80	10-50	<10
Cefonicid	Renal	4-5	50-60	-	.5-2 gm q24h	8-25 mg/kg q24h	4-15 mg/kg q24-48h	3-15 mg/kg q3-5d
Cefoperazone	Gut	1.9-2.5	2-2.5	-	1-2 gm q 6-12h	Usual	Usual	Usual
Ceforanide	Renal	3	20-40	-	0.5-1 gm q12h	Usual	0.5-1 gm q24h	0.5-1 gm q48-72h
Cefotaxime	Renal	1.1	3	-	1-2 gm q4-6h	Usual	1-2 gm q6-12h	1-2 gm q12h
Cefotetan	Renal	3-4	12-30	-	1-2 gm q12h	Usual	1-2 gm q24h	1-2 gm q48h
Cefoxitin	Renal	0.7	13-22	-	1-2 gm q6-8h	1-2 gm q8-12h	1-2 gm q12-24h	0.5-1 gm q12-48h
Ceftazidime	Renal	1.5-2	15-25	-	1-2 gm q8-12h	Usual	1 gm q12-24h	0.5 gm q24-48h
Ceftizoxime	Renal	1.4-1.8	25-35	-	1-3 gm q6-8h	0.5-1.5 gm q8h	.25-1 gm q12h	.25 gm q24h
Ceftriaxone	Renal & Gut	6-9	12-15	-	0.5-1 gm q12-24h	Usual	Usual	Usual
Cefuroxime	Renal	1.3-1.7	20	-	.75-1.5 gm q8h	Usual	0.75-1.5 gm q8-12h	0.75 gm q24h

(continued)

Drug	Major excretory route	Half life (hr) Normal	Anuria	Usual regimen Oral	Parenteral	Maintenance regimen renal failure Glomerular filtration rate in mL/min 50-80	10-50	< 10
Cefuroxime axetil	Renal	1.2	20	250 mg q12h	-	Usual	Usual	250 mg q 24h
Cephalexin	Renal	0.9	5-30	0.25-1.0 gm q6h	-	Usual	0.25-1.0 gm q8-12h	0.25-1 gm q24-48h
Cephalothin	Renal	0.5-0.9	3-8	-	.5-2 gm q4-6h	Usual	1.0-1.5 gm q6h	.5 gm q8h
Cephapirin	Renal	0.6-.9	2.4	-	0.5-2 gm q4-6h	0.5-2 gm q6h	0.5-2 gm q8h	0.5-2 gm q12h
Cephradine	Renal	.7-1	8-15	0.25-1.0 gm q6h -	- 0.5-2 gm q4-6h	Usual 0.5-1 gm q6h	0.5 gm q6h 0.5-1 gm q6-24h	0.25 gm q12h 0.5-1 gm q24-72h
Chloramphenicol	Hepatic	2.5	3-7	0.25-0.75 gm q6h	.25-1 gm q6h	Usual	Usual	Usual
Chloroquine	Renal & metabolized	48-120	?	300-600 mg po qd	-	Usual	Usual	150-300 mg po qd
Cinoxacin	Renal	1.5	8.5	.25-.5 gm q12h	-	.25 gm q8h	.25 gm q12h	.25 gm q24h
Ciprofloxacin	Renal & hepatic	4	5-10	.25-.75 gm q12h	-	Usual	.25-.5 gm q12h	.25-.5 gm q18h
Clindamycin	Hepatic	2-2.5	2-3.5	150-300 mg q6h	300-900 mg q6-8h	Usual	Usual	Usual

(continued)

Drug	Major excretory route	Half life (hr) Normal	Half life (hr) Anuria	Usual regimen Oral	Usual regimen Parenteral	Maintenance regimen renal failure Glomerular filtration rate in mL/min 50-80	10-50	< 10
Clofazimine	Hepatic	8 days	8 days	50 mg qd 100 mg tid	-	Usual	Usual	Usual
Cloxacillin	Renal	0.5	0.8	0.5-1.0 gm q6h	-	Usual	Usual	Usual
Colistin	Renal	3-8	10-20	-	1.5 mg/kg q6-12h	2.5-3.8 mg/kg/day	1.5-2.5 mg/kg q24-36h	.6 mg/kg q24h
Cycloserine	Renal	8-12	?	250-500 mg bid	-	Usual	250-500 mg qd	250 mg qd
Dapsone	Hepatic metabolism	30	slight	50-100 mg/day	-	Usual	Usual	(No data)
Dicloxacillin	Renal	0.5-0.9	1-1.6	0.25-0.5 gm q6h	-	Usual	Usual	Usual
Doxycycline	Renal	14-25	15-36	100 mg bid	100 mg bid	Usual	Usual	Usual
Erythromycin	Hepatic	1.2-2.6	4-6	.25-.5 gm q6h	1 gm q6h	Usual	Usual	Usual
Ethambutol	Renal	3-4	8	15-25 mg/kg q24h	-	15 mg/kg q24h	15 mg/kg q24-36h	15 mg/kg q48h
Ethionamide	Metabolized	4	8	.5-1 gm/day 1-3 doses	-	Usual	Usual	5 mg/kg q24h
Flucytosine	Renal	3-6	70	37 mg/kg q6h	-	Usual	37 mg/kg q12-24 h	Not recommended

36

(continued)

Drug	Major excretory route	Half life (hr) Normal	Anuria	Usual regimen Oral	Parenteral	Maintenance regimen renal failure Glomerular filtration rate in mL/min 50-80	10-50	< 10
Ganciclovir (induction doses)	Renal	1.5-3	↑↑	-	5.0 mg/kg IV bid	2.5 mg/kg bid	2.5 mg/kg qd	1.5 mg/kg qd
Gentamicin	Renal	2	48	-	1.7 mg/kg q8h	See pg 30,31		
Griseofulvin microsize	Hepatic metabolism	24	24	.5-1 gm q d	-	Usual	Usual	Usual
ultramicrosize	(Same)	(Same)	(Same)	.33-.66 gm q d	-	Usual	Usual	Usual
Imipenem	Renal	.8-1	3.5	-	0.5-1 gm q6h	0.5 gm q6-8h	0.5 gm q8-12h	0.25-0.5 mg q12h
Isoniazid	Hepatic	0.5-4	2-10	300 mg q24h	300 mg q24h	Usual	Usual	Slow acetylators 1/2 dose
Kanamycin	Renal	2-3	27-30	-	7.5 mg/kg	See pg 30,31		
Ketoconazole	Hepatic metabolism	1-4	1-4	200-400 mg q12-24h	-	Usual	Usual	Usual
Methenamine hippurate	Renal	3-6	?	1 gm q12h	-	Usual	Avoid	Avoid
mandelate	Renal	3-6	?	1 gm q12h	-	Usual	Avoid	Avoid
Methicillin	Renal (hepatic)	0.5	4	-	1-2 gm q4-6h	1-2 gm q6h	1-2 gm q8h	1-2 gm q12h
Metronidazole	Hepatic	6-14	8-15	.25-7.5 gm tid	.5 gm q6h	Usual	Usual	Usual **(continued)**

Drug	Major excretory route	Half life (hr) Normal	Half life (hr) Anuria	Usual regimen Oral	Usual regimen Parenteral	Maintenance regimen renal failure Glomerular filtration rate in mL/min 50-80	10-50	<10
Mezlocillin	Renal	1	1.5	-	3-4 gm q4-6h	Usual	3 gm q8h	2 gm q8h
Miconazole	Hepatic	0.5-1	0.5-1	-	0.4-1.2 gm q8h	Usual	Usual	Usual
Minocycline	Hepatic & metabolized	11-26	17-30	100 mg q12h	100 mg q12h	Usual	Usual	Usual or sl decrease
Moxalactam	Renal	2	20	-	1-4 gm q8-12h	3 gm q8h	2-3 gm q12h	1 gm 12-24h
Nafcillin	Hepatic metabolism	0.5	1.2	0.5-1 gm q6h	0.5-2 gm q4-6h	Usual	Usual	Usual
Nalidixic acid	Renal & metabolized	1.5	21	1 gm q6h	-	Usual	Usual	Avoid
Netilmicin	Renal	2.5	35	-	2.0 mg/kg q8h	See pg 30,31		
Nitrofurantoin	Renal	0.3	1	50-100 mg q6-8h	-	Usual	Avoid	Avoid
Norfloxacin	Renal & metabolized	3.5	8	400 mg bid	-	Usual	400 mg qd	400 mg qd
Nystatin	Not absorbed	-	-	.4-1 mil units 3-5 x daily	-	Usual	Usual	Usual

38

(continued)

Drug	Major excretory route	Half life (hr) Normal	Anuria	Usual regimen Oral	Parenteral	Maintenance regimen renal failure Glomerular filtration rate in mL/min 50-80	10-50	< 10
Oxacillin	Renal	0.5	1	0.5-1 gm q6h	0.5-2 gm q4-6h	Usual	Usual	Usual
Penicillin G crystalline	Renal	0.5	7-10	0.4-0.8 mil units q6h	1-4 mil units q4-6h	Usual	Usual	½ usual dose
procaine	Renal	24	^	-	0.6-1.2 mil units IM q12h	Usual	Usual	Usual
benzathine	Renal	days	↑	-	0.6-1.2 mil units IM	Usual	Usual	Usual
V	Renal	0.5	7-10	0.4-0.8 mil units q6h	-	Usual	Usual	Usual
Pentamidine	Renal	1-9	?	-	4 mg/kg q24h	Usual	4 mg/kg q24-36h	4 mg/kg q48h
Piperacillin	Renal	1.0	3.0	-	3-4 gm q4-6h	Usual	3 gm q8h	3 gm q12h
Polymyxin B	Renal	6	48	-	.8-1.2 gm IV q12h	1-1.5 mg/kg qd	1-1.5 mg/kg q2-3d	1 mg/kg q5-7d

(continued)

Drug	Major excretory route	Half life (hr) Normal	Anuria	Usual regimen Oral	Parenteral	Maintenance regimen renal failure Glomerular filtration rate in mL/min 50-80	10-50	< 10
Praziquantel	Hepatic metabolism	0.8-1.5	?	10-25 mg/kg tid	-	Usual	Usual	Usual
Pyrazinamide	Metabolized	10-16	?	15-35 mg/kg daily	-	Usual	Usual	12-20 mg/kg/day
Pyrimethamine	Nonrenal	1.5-5 days	?	25 mg/day	-	Usual	Usual	Usual
Quinine	Hepatic metabolism	5-16	?	650 mg tid	7.5-10 mg/kg q8h	Usual	I 8-12h	I 24h
Rifampin	Hepatic	2-5	2-5	600 mg/day	600 mg/day	Usual	Usual	Usual
Spectinomycin	Renal	1-3	?	-	2 gm IM/day	Usual	Usual	Usual
Streptomycin	Renal	2.5	100-110	-	500 mg q12h	7.5 mg/kg q24h	7.5 mg/kg q24-72h	7.5 mg/kg q72-96h
Sulfadiazine	Renal	17	?	0.5-1.5 gm q4-6h	-	Usual	0.5-1.5 gm q8-12h	0.5-1.5 gm q12-24h
				-	30-50 mg/kg q6-8h	Usual	30-50 mg/kg q 12-18h	30-50 mg/kg q18-24h
Sulfisoxazole	Renal	3-7	6-12	1-2 gm q6h	-	Usual	1 gm q 8-12h	1 gm q 12-24h
Tetracycline	Renal	8	50-100	.25-.5 gm q6h	.5-1 gm q12h	Usual	Use doxycycline **(continued)**	

Drug	Major excretory route	Half life (hr) Normal	Half life (hr) Anuria	Usual regimen Oral	Usual regimen Parenteral	Maintenance regimen renal failure Glomerular filtration rate in mL/min 50-80	10-50	<10
Ticarcillin	Renal	1-1.5	16	-	3 gm q4h	Usual	2-3 gm q 6-8 h	2 gm q12h
Ticarcillin + clavulanic acid	Renal	1-1.5	16	-	3 gm q4h	Usual	2-3 gm q6-8h	2 gm q12h
Tobramycin	Renal	2.5	56	-	1.7 mg/kg q8h	See pg 30,31		
Trimethoprim	Renal	8-15	24	100 mg q12h	-	Usual	100 mg q18-24h	Avoid
Trimethoprim-sulfamethoxazole	Renal	T:8-15 S:7-12	T:24 S:22-50	2-4 tabs/d or 1-2 DS/day	-	Usual	Half dose	1 tab bid
					3-5 mg/kg q6-12h	3-5 mg/kg q18h	3-5 mg/kg q24h	Avoid
Vancomycin	Renal	6-8	200-250	PO: .125-.5 gm q6h	15 mg/kg q12h	PO: usual dose IV: 1 gm q24h	IV: 1 gm q3-10d	0.125 mg po IV: 1 gm q5-10d
Vidarabine	Renal	1.5		-	15 mg/kg/ day	Usual	Usual	10 mg/kg/ day
Zidovudine AZT	Hepatic metabolism	1	?	100-200 mg q4h	-	Usual	Usual	Usual

USE OF ANTIMICROBIAL AGENTS IN HEPATIC DISEASE

Many antimicrobial agents are metabolized by the liver and/or excreted via the biliary tract. Nevertheless, relatively few require dose modifications in hepatic disease; with the exceptions, doses are usually modified only if there is concurrent renal failure and/or the liver disease is either acute or is associated with severe hepatic failure as indicated by ascites or jaundice. The following recommendations are adopted from "Drug Information 88", American Hospital Formulary Service, Amer Soc Hosp Pharmacists, Bethesda, Md 1988

Agent: Recommended dose modification

Aztreonam: Some recommend a dose reduction of 20-25%.

Carbenicillin: Maximum of 2 gm/day for patients with severe renal and hepatic insufficiency.

Cefoperazone: Maximum dose is 4 gm/day; if higher monitor levels; with coexisting renal impairment maximum dose is 1-2 gm/day.

Ceftriaxone: Maximum daily dose of 2 gm with severe hepatic and renal impairment.

Chloramphenicol: Use with caution with renal and/or hepatic failure; monitor serum levels to achieve levels of 5-20 μg/mL.

Clindamycin: Dose reduction recommended only for severe hepatic failure.

Isoniazid: Use with caution and monitor hepatic function for mild-moderate hepatic disease; acute liver disease or history of INH-associated hepatic injury is contraindicated to INH.

Mezlocillin: Reduce dose by 50% or double the dosing interval.

Nafcillin: Metabolized by liver and largely eliminated in bile; nevertheless, dose modifications are suggested only for combined hepatic and renal failure.

Penicillin G: Dose reduction recommended for hepatic failure only when accompanied by renal failure.

Rifampin: Induces hepatic enzymes responsible for inactivating methadone, corticosteroids, oral anticoagulants, oral antidiabetic agents, digitalis, quinidine, cyclosporine, estrogens, oral contraceptives and chloramphenicol. Concurrent use of these drugs with rifampin and use of rifampin in patients with prior liver disease requires careful review.

Ticarcillin: For patients with hepatic dysfunction and creatinine clearance < 10 mL/min, give 2 gm IV/day in one or two doses.

Ticarcillin/Clavulanate K: For patients with hepatic dysfunction and creatinine clearance < 10 mL/min give usual loading dose (3.1 gm) followed by 2 gm once daily.

ADVERSE REACTIONS TO ANTIMICROBIAL AGENTS

A. Adverse Reactions by Class

	Frequent	Occasional	Rare
Acyclovir	Irritation at infusion site; renal toxicity (esp with rapid IV infusion, prior renal disease and other nephrotoxic drugs); headache	Rash; nausea; diarrhea; vertigo (oral); marrow suppression; metabolic encephalopathy; abnormal liver function tests	CNS-agitation, lethargy, disorientation, transient hemiparesis, seizures
Amantadine	Insomnia, lethargy, dizziness, inability to concentrate	CNS-depression, confusion, slurred speech; congestive heart failure; GI intolerance, rash	CNS-psychosis, convulsions; eczematoid dermatitis; photosensitivity; oculogyric episodes; orthostatic hypotension; peripheral edema; bone marrow suppression
Aminoglycosides Tobramycin Gentamicin Amikacin Netilmicin Kanamycin	Renal failure	Vestibular and auditory damage	Fever; rash; blurred vision; neuromuscular blockage; eosinophilia
Aminosalicylic acid (PAS)	GI intolerance	Liver damage; allergic reactions; thyroid enlargement	Acidosis; vasculitis; hypoglycemia (diabetes); hypokalemia; encephalopathy; decreased prothrombin activity; myalgias; renal damage; gastric hemorrhage **(continued)**

	Frequent	Occasional	Rare
Amoxicillin + clavulanic acid	(Similar to amoxicillin - See penicillins)		
Amphotericin B	Renal damage; hypokalemia; anemia; phlebitis and pain at injection site; nausea; vomiting; metallic taste; fever; chills; headache	Hypomagnesemia	Hypotension; rash; pruritis; blurred vision; peripheral neuropathy; convulsions; hemorrhagic gastroenteritis; arrhythmias; diabetes insipidis; hearing loss; pulmonary edema; anaphylaxis; acute hepatic failure; eosinophilia; leukopenia; thrombocytopenia
Ampicillin + sulbactam	Similar to those for ampicillin alone (See penicillins)		
Aztreonam	Eosinophilia	Phlebitis at infusion site; rash; diarrhea, nausea; eosinophilia; abnormal liver function tests	Thrombocytopenia; colitis; hypotension; unusual taste; seizures; chills
Bacitracin	Nephrotoxicity (proteinuria, oliguria, azotemia); pain with IM use		Rash; blood dyscrasias
Capreomycin	Renal damage (tubular necrosis esp in patients with prior renal damage	Ototoxicity (vestibular and auditory); electrolyte abnormalities; pain, induration and sterile abscesses at injection sites	Allergic rections; leukopenia; leukocytosis; neuromuscular blockage (large IV doses-reversed with neostigmine); hypersensitivity reactions **(continued)**

44

	Frequent	Occasional	Rare
Cephalosporins	Phlebitis at infusion sites; diarrhea (esp cefoperazone); pain at IM injection sites (less with cefazolin)	Allergic reactions (anaphylaxis rare); diarrhea and colitis; hypo-prothrombinemia (cefamandole, cefoperazone, moxalactam and cefotetan); platelet dysfunction (moxalactam); eosinophilia; positive Coombs' test	Hemolytic anemia; interstitial nephritis (cephalothin); hepatic dysfunction; convulsions (high dose with renal failure); neutropenia; thrombocytopenia
Chloramphenicol		GI intolerance (oral); marrow suppression (dose related)	Fatal aplastic anemia; fever; allergic reactions; peripheral neuropathy; optic neuritis
Chloroquine		Visual disturbances (related to dose and duration of treatment); GI intolerance; pruritis	CNS-headache, confusion, psychosis; peripheral neuropathy; cardiac toxicity; hemolysis (G-6-PD deficiency); marrow suppression
Ciprofloxacin	See quinolones		
Clindamycin	Diarrhea	Rash; colitis; GI intolerance (oral)	Blood dyscrasias; hepatic damage; neutropenia; neuromuscular blockage; eosinophilia; fever; metallic taste; phlebitis at IV infusion sites
Clofazimine	Ichthyosis; discoloration of skin, cornea, retina and urine (with prolonged use); GI intolerance	Persistent abdominal pain, diarrhea and weight loss (high dose over 3 months); dry, burning, irritated eyes	Bowel obstruction; GI bleeding; splenic infarction; eosinophilic enteritis; vision loss
Colistimethate	(See Polymyxins)		

(continued)

	Frequent	Occasional	Rare
Cycloserine	CNS-anxiety, confusion depression, somnolence, disorientation, headache, hallucinations, tremor, hyperreflexia, increased CSF protein and pressure (dose related and reversible)	Liver damage; malabsorption; peripheral neuropathy; folate deficiency; anemia	Coma; seizures (contra-indicated in epileptics); hypersensitivity reactions; heart failure, arrhythmias
Dapsone	Rash; headache (transient); GI intolerance; infectious mono-like syndrome	Blood dyscrasias (methemoglobulinemia and sulfahemoglobinemia); hemolytic anemia; nephrotic syndrome; allergic reactions; insomnia; irritability; uncoordinated speech; agitation; psychosis	Hypoalbuminemia; epidermal necrolysis; optic atrophy; agranulocytosis
Emetine	Arrhythmias; precordial pain; muscle weakness; phlebitis	Diarrhea; vomiting; neuropathy; heart failure	
Erythromycins	GI intolerance (oral-dose related); phlebitis (IV)	Diarrhea; stomatitis; cholestatic hepatitis (esp estolate-reversible); phlebitis (IV administration); generalized rash	Allergic reactions; colitis; hemolytic anemia; reversible ototoxicity (esp high dose and renal failure)
Ethambutol		Optic neuritis; allergic reactions; GI intolerance; confusion; precipitation of acute gout	Peripheral neuropathy; thrombocytopenia; toxic epidermal necrolysis; lichenoid skin rash **(continued)**

46

	Frequent	Occasional	Rare
Ethionamide	GI intolerance (improved with antacids); depression	Allergic reactions; peripheral neuropathy; liver damage; gynecomastia; menstrual irregularity	Optic neuritis; gouty arthritis; hypothyroidism; impotence; thyroid enlargement; poor diabetic control; rash; hepatitis
Flucytosine	GI intolerance (including nausea, vomiting, diarrhea and ulcerative colitis)	Rash; liver damage (dose related); marrow suppression (dose related, esp with renal failure or concurrent amphotericin); confusion	Hallucinations; eosinophilia; granulocytosis
Furazolidone	GI intolerance	Allergic reactions; pulmonary infiltrates; headache	Hemolytic anemia (G-6-PD deficiency); hypotension; polyneuropathy; hypoglycemia; agranulocytosis
Ganciclovir (DHPG)	Neutropenia	Thrombocytopenia; rash; hypotension; nausea; vomiting; changes in mental status; renal failure; abnormal liver functions tests; headache; fever	Psychosis; neuropathy; impaired reproductive function (?); carcinogenic in animals (? significance); hearing loss; GI bleeding or perforation; myocardiopathy
Griseofulvin	Headache (often resolves with continued treatment)	Photosensitivity	GI disturbance; allergic reactions; paresthesias; exacerbation of lupus; liver damage; lymphadenopathy; blood dyscrasias; thrush; transient hearing loss; fatigue; dizziness; insomnia; psychosis **(continued)**

47

	Frequent	Occasional	Rare
Imipenem		Phlebitis at infusion sites; allergic reactions; nausea, vomiting and diarrhea; eosinophilia; hepatotoxicity (transient)	Seizures; myoclonus; colitis; bone marrow suppression; renal toxicity
Isoniazid	Hepatitis (patients over 35 yrs and usually reversible)	Allergic reactions; fever; peripheral neuropathy (reduce with pyridoxine)	CNS-optic neuritis, psychosis, convulsions, toxic encephalopathy, twitching, coma; blood dyscrasias; hyperglycemia; lupus-like syndrome; keratitis; pellagra-like rash
Ketoconazole	GI intolerance (dose related)	Hepatic toxicity (usually reversible); endocrine-decreased steroid and testosterone synthesis with impotence, gynecomastia, reduced libido, menstrual abnormalities (prolonged use); headache, dizziness; asthenia; pruritis; rash	Fatal hepatic necrosis; anaphylaxis; lethargy; arthralgias; fever; marrow suppression
Methenamine		GI intolerance; dysuria (reduced dose or acidification)	Allergic reactions; edema; tinnitus; muscle cramps
Metronidazole	GI intolerance; metallic taste; headache	Peripheral neuropathy (prolonged use - reversible); phlebitis at injection sites; Antabuse-like reaction	Seizures; ataxic encephalitis; colitis; leukopenia; dysuria; pancreatitis; allergic reactions; mutagenic in Ames test (significance unknown) **(continued)**

48

	Frequent	Occasional	Rare
Miconazole		Phlebitis at injections sites; chills; pruritis; rash; dizziness; blurred vision; hyperlipidemia; nausea; vomiting; hyponatremia	Marrow suppression - anemia and thrombocytopenia; renal damage; anaphylaxis; psychosis; cardiac arrest
Nalidixic acid	(See quinolones)		
Nitrofurantoin	GI intolerance	Hypersensitivity reactions; pulmonary infiltrates (acute, subacute or chronic; $\pm$ fever, eosinophilia, rash or lupus-like reaction)	Peripheral neuropathy; hepatitis; hemolytic anemia (G-6-PD deficiency); lactic acidosis; parotitis; pancreatitis
Nystatin		GI intolerance	Allergic reactions
Penicillins	Hypersensitivity reactions; rash (esp ampicillin and amoxicillin); diarrhea (esp ampicillin)	GI intolerance (oral agents); fever; Coombs' test positive; phlebitis at infusion sites and sterile abscesses at IM sites; Jarisch-Herxheimer reaction (syphilis or other spirochetal infections)	Anaphylaxis; leukopenia, thrombocytopenia; colitis (esp ampicillin); hepatic damage; renal damage; CNS-seizures, twitching (high doses in patients with renal failure); hyperkalemia (K penicillin G infusion); abnormal platelet aggregation with bleeding diathesis (carbenicillin and ticarcillin)
Pentamidine	Nephrotoxicity; GI intolerance	Hypotension; hypoglycemia; rash (including Stevens-Johnson syndrome); marrow suppression (common in AIDS patients)	Increased liver function tests; pancreatitis; bronchospasm (inhalation); hyperglycemia, insulin-dependent diabetes **(continued)**

49

	Frequent	Occasional	Rare
Polymyxins Colistimethate	Pain and phlebitis at injection sites; neurotoxicity (ataxia, paresthesias); nephrotoxicity		Allergic reactions; neuromuscular blockade
Primaquine		Hemolytic anemia (G-6-PD deficiency); GI intolerance	Headache; pruritis
Pyrazinamide		Hepatitis; hyperuricemia; arthralgias; GI intolerance	Rash; fever; porphyria; photosensitivity
Pyrimethamine		Folic acid deficiency with megaloblastic anemia and pancytopenia (dose related and reversed with leucovorin); allergic reactions	CNS-ataxia, tremors, seizures (dose related), fatigue
Quinine		GI intolerance; cinchonism (tinnitis, headache, visual disturbances); hemolytic anemia (G-6-PD deficiency)	Arrhythmias; hypotension with rapid IV infusion; hypoglycemia; hepatitis; thrombocytopenia
Quinolones	(Animal studies show arthropathies in weight bearing joints of immature animals; significance in humans is not known, but this class is considered contraindicated in children and pregnancy)	GI intolerance; CNS-headache, malaise, insomnia, dizziness; allergic reactions	Papilledema; nystagmus; visual disturbances; diarrhea; abnormal liver function tests; marrow suppression; photosensitivity

50

(continued)

	Frequent	Occasional	Rare
Rifampin	Orange discoloration of urine, tears (contact lens), sweat	Hepatitis; GI intolerance; hypersensitivity reactions; increases hepatic metabolism of steroids to increase steroid requirement in adrenal insufficiency and require alternative to birth control meds; flu-like syndrome with intermittent use	Thrombocytopenia; leukopenia; eosinophilia; renal damage; proximal myelopathy
Spectinomycin		Pain at injection site; urticaria; fever; insomnia; dizziness; nausea; headache	Anaphylaxis; fever; anemia; renal failure and abnormal liver function tests (multiple doses)
Sulfonamides	Allergic reactions- rash, pruritis, fever	Periarteritis nodosum, lupus, Stevens-Johnson syndrome, serum sickness; crystalluria with renal damage, urolithiasis and oliguria; GI intolerance; photosensitivity	Myocarditis; psychosis, neuropathy, dizziness, depression; hemolytic anemia (G-6-PD deficiency); marrow suppression; agranulocytosis

Tetracyclines
  Tetracycline HCl
  Demeclocycline
  Doxycycline
  Minocycline
	GI intolerance (dose-related); stains and deforms teeth in children up to 8 yrs; vertigo (minocycline); negative nitrogen balance and increased azotemia with renal failure (except doxycycline); vaginitis	Hepatotoxicity (dose-related, esp pregnant women); esophageal ulcerations; diarrhea; Candidiasis (thrush and vaginitis); photosensitivity (esp demeclocycline); phlebitis with IV treatment and pain with IM injection	Malabsorption; allergic reactions; visual disturbances; aggravation of myasthenia; hemolytic anemia; colitis

(continued)

	Frequent	Occasional	Rare
Ticarcillin + clavulanic acid	Similar to those for ticarcillin alone (See penicillins)		
Trimethoprim	GI intolerance (dose-related); rash	Marrow-megaloblastic anemia, neutropenia, thrombocytopenia	Pancytopenia
Trimethoprim-sulfamethoxazole	Fever, leukopenia, rash (AIDS patients); reactions noted above for sulfonamides and trimethoprim		
Vancomycin	Phlebitis at injection sites	"Red-man syndrome" (flushing over chest and face) or hypotension (infusion too rapid); rash; fever; neutropenia; eosinophilia; allergic reactions with rash	Anaphylaxis; ototoxicity and nephrotoxicity (dose related); peripheral neuropathy; marrow suppression
Vidarabine		GI intolerance; phlebitis at infusion site; fluid overload	Blood dyscrasias; CNS-confusion and neurologic deterioration (esp with renal failure)
Zidovudine (AZT, Retrovir)	Anemia; leukopenia	Headache; malaise; insomia; myalgias; myopathy	Neurotoxicity - headache, confusion, aphasia, twitching, seizures (reversible); allergy - anaphylaxis, urticaria, wheezing

B. Penicillin Allergy (Adapted from The Medical Letter 30:77,1988)

Cross reactions

1. Allergy to one penicillin indicates allergy to all.

2. Persons allergic to penicillins may have allergic reactions to cephalosporins or imipenem.

3. There is no apparent cross reaction with aztreonam.

Tests for penicillin allergy

1. Negative tests with two-test preparations are $\geq 99\%$ effective in predicting safety from IgE mediated response.

2. Preparations

   a. Penicilloyl-polylysine (Pre-Pen).

   b. "Minor determinants" not commercially available; alternative is aqueous penicillin G, but 25% who react with minor determinants do not test positive with penicillin G.

3. Technique: Two preparations are given in separate injection sites with histamine (positive control) and diluent (negative control).

   a. "Prick test": Small drop on skin and then skin indentation with needle bevel at 30° angle.

   b. If no reaction (wheal $\geq$ 5mm) in 15 minutes: Intradermal injection using 27 gauge needle to produce a detectable bleb (0.01-0.02 ml).

   c. Positive test is wheal $\geq$ 5mm; negative test is equivalent to negative control; all other results are indeterminant.

Test doses: Skin test negative: First dose is 1,000-2,000 units (3-5 mg) penicillin IV or 1-2 mg po with observation for 1 hr before proceeding to larger dose. Proceed to full doses or incremental doses depending on the history.

Desensitization

1. Perform only in hospital with constant supervision, IV in place and supportive equipment and drugs readily available.

2. Give 1 unit penicillin IV and then double dose at 15 minute intervals or increase dose 10-fold at 20-30 minute intervals.

C. Adverse Reactions during Pregnancy (Adapted from Drug Evaluations, 6th Edition, AMA, Chicago, 1986, pp 44-46)

Agent	1st trimester (Embryonic development)	2nd & 3rd trimester (Fetal development)	Labor-delivery
Antibacterial agents			
Aminoglycosides	8th nerve damage**	8th nerve damage**	-
Chloramphenicol	-	Gray-baby syndrome*	Gray-baby syndrome*
Dapsone	-	-	Carcinogenic*** Hemolytic reactions
Streptomycin	8th nerve damage multiple defects, micromelia*	8th nerve damage*	-
Sulfamethoxazole-trimethoprim	Malformations****	-	-
Sulfonamides	-	Hyperbilirubinemia* Hemolytic anemia*	Hyperbilirubinemia* Hemolytic anemia*
Nitrofurantoin	-	-	Hyperbilirubinemia*
Tetracycline	Inhibit bone growth* Micromelia** Syndactyly**	Stain deciduous teeth* Inhibit bone growth* Enamel hypoplasia**	-
Metronidazole	Tumors***	-	-
Antimalarial agents			
Quinine	Malformations, abortions, 8th nerve damage*	Deafness Thrombocytopenia	-
Chloroquine	8th nerve damage**	8th nerve damage**	-
Antituberculous agents			
Rifampin	CNS effects***	-	-
Isoniazid	CNS effects***	-	-
Streptomycin (see above)			

* Generally well documented in man
** Suspected in man
*** Documented in animals only
**** Questionable effects in man

54

D. Relative Safety during Pregnancy (Classification according to Medical Letter 29:61-64,1987)

	Probably safe	Caution	Contraindicated
Antibacterial agents	Aztreonam Cephalosporins Erythromycins (not estolate) Methenamine Penicillins Spectinomycin	Aminoglycosides Chloramphenicol Clindamycin Dapsone Imipenem Metronidazole Nitrofurantoin Sulfonamides Trimethoprim Trimethoprim-sulfa Vancomycin	Cinoxacin Ciprofloxacin Erythromycin (estolate) Nalidixic acid Norfloxacin Tetracyclines
Antifungal agents	Nystatin	Amphotericin B Flucytosine Ketoconazole Miconazole	Griseofulvin
Antiviral agents		Acyclovir Vidarabine Zidovudine (Retrovir, AZT)	Amantadine Ribavirin
Antituberculosis agents		Capreomycin Cycloserine Ethambutol Ethionamide Isoniazid Pyrazinamide Rifampin Streptomycin	
Antiparasitic agents	Chloroquine Niclosamide Paromycin Praziquantel Pyrethrins	Diloxanide Furazolidone Iodoquinol Mebendazole Metronidazole Pentamidine Piperazine Pyrimethamine Pyrimethamine- sulfadoxine Quinacrine Quinine Suramin Thiabendazole	Emetine Lindane

DRUG INTERACTIONS
(Adapted from Drug Evaluations 6th Edition, AMA, Chicago 1986, pp 32-38)

Drug	Interacting agent	Effect	Comment
Alcohol	Metronidazole Cefamandole Cefoperazone Moxalactam & Cefotetan	Disulfiram-like reaction (facial flush, sweating, nausea, tachycardia)	Warn patient to limit or avoid alcohol
Aminoglycosides	Cephalothin & Ethacrynic acid	Additive ototoxicity	Avoid, especially when concurrent renal damage; monitor hearing
Antipseudomonad penicillins	Decreases aminoglycoside activity in patients with renal failure		
Anticoagulants (oral)	Metronidazole Sulfonamides Moxalactam & Cefamandole	Enhanced anticoagulant activity	Monitor prothrombin time
	Griseofulvin & Rifampin	Decreased anticoagulant activity	
Cyclosporin	Ketoconazole Erythromycin	Enhanced cyclosporin activity with renal or CNS toxicity	Inhibits cytochrome P-450 enzymes
	Rifampin	Decreased cyclosporin activity	Induction of hepatic enzymes
	Aminoglycosides, Amphotericin B	Renal insufficiency	Additive nephrotoxicity
Digitalis preparations	Erythromycin & Tetracycline, etc	Digitalis toxicity	Antibiotics active versus Eubacterium in the gut are the additional theoretic causes; mechanism is loss of digitalis reducing enzymes in gut flora; ~10% are susceptible

56

Drug	Interacting agent	Effect	Comment
Disulfiram	Metronidazole	Acute psychoses	
Oral contraceptives	Ampicillin & Tetracycline	Decreased contraceptive activity	Interfere with enterohepatic circulation of estrogens
	Rifampin	Decreased contraceptive activity	Enhance estrogen metabolism
Phenytoin	Chloramphenicol Isoniazid Trimethoprim & Sulfonamides	Increased phenytoin concentration	
Quinidine	Rifampin	Decreased quinidine activity	Induction of hepatic enzymes
Sulfonylureas	Chloramphenicol & Sulfonamides	Increased hypoglycemic activity	Inhibit hepatic metabolism
Tetracyclines	Antacids Calcium, iron and Mg containing compounds	Decreased bioavailability of tetracyclines	Antacids, calcium and magnesium containing cpds chelate tetracyclines other than doxycycline; Fe cpds reduce bioavailability of all tetracyclines

57

ADULT IMMUNIZATION
Recommendations of the Advisory Committee on Immunization Practices
(MMWR 33:S1–S37,1984; Ann Intern Med 108:616,1988)

Patient category	Vaccine	Comment
Age 18–24 yrs	Td*	Booster every 10 yrs for those who completed primary series**
	Measles***	Persons vaccinated 1963–1967 with inactivated vaccine or vaccine of unknown type should be revaccinated with live virus vaccine
	Mumps***	Especially susceptible males
	Rubella***	Especially susceptible females; pregnancy is contraindication
25–64 yrs	Td*, Mumps***	As above
	Measles**	Primarily non-immune persons born after 1956
	Rubella***	Principally females up to 45 yrs with childbearing potential
> 65 yrs	Td*	As above
	Influenza	Annually
	Pneumococcal	Single dose (efficacy not established) **(continued)**

Patient category	Vaccine	Comment
Occupation, setting or life style		
Health care workers	Hepatitis B	Personnel having contact with blood or blood products
	Rubella	Personnel who are not immune and at risk for exposure to rubella or who have contact with pregnant patients***
	Measles	Personnel who are not immune and born after 1956 and have contact with measles cases***
	Poliovirus	Hospital and laboratory personnel who are not immune (proof of completing primary series) and who are at risk of contacting patients or specimens with wild poliovirus should receive inactivated poliovirus vaccine (IPV)
Homosexual men	Hepatitis B	Prevaccination serologic screening advocated
IV drug abusers	Hepatitis B	As above
Residents of institutions for mentally retarded	Hepatitis B	New admissions should be vaccinated. Current residents: prevaccination serologic screening advocated
Foreign students, immigrants and refugees	Td*, measles, rubella	Use age guidelines above for persons who cannot document prior vaccination or laboratory evidence of immunity
	Poliovirus	Recommended only for persons under 18 yrs **(continued)**

Patient category	Vaccine	Comment
Pregnancy		Delay any vaccine or toxoid to second or third trimester when possible; avoid live virus vaccines****
	Td*	If not previously vaccinated give 2 doses properly spaced (4 wks) with 3rd dose at 6-12 months; boost if 10 years or more since primary series
	Oral poliovirus vaccine	Advised if exposure is imminent
	Yellow fever	Advised if exposure is imminent; if only reason is travel requirement, attempt to use waiver letter
	Rubella	Give postpartum if immunity not established
Hemodialysis patients	Hepatitis B	Double dose suggested, prevaccination serologic screening advocated
	Influenza	
	Pneumococcal vaccine	
Splenic dysfunction or asplenia	Pneumococcal vaccine Influenza	Give two weeks before elective splenectomy
Factor VIII and IX deficiencies	Hepatitis B	Prevaccination serologic screening advocated
Chronic alcoholism	Pneumococcal vaccine	

(continued)

Patient category	Vaccine	Comment
Veterinarians and animal handlers	Rabies vaccine (HDCV)	Persons at risk for rabies exposure. Continued risk: Booster dose of HDCV every 2 yrs or serology showing titer < 5 by rapid fluorescent - focus inhibition test
Compromised host (Leukemia, lymphoma, immunosuppressive treatment)	Pneumococcal vaccine Influenza	Avoid live virus vaccines**** Ability to respond after immunosuppressive treatment is estimated at 3-12 months
AIDS	Influenza Pneumococcal vaccine	
Travelers		For travelers to developed countries (Canada, Europe, Japan, Australia and New Zealand) the risk of developing vaccine preventable disease is no greater than traveling in the U.S.
	Polio	Unimmunized travelers to underdeveloped countries should receive 2 doses of IVP one month apart, and preferrably complete the primary series before travel. If not possible, give a single dose of OPV. For vaccinated travelers, complete the series or give a single dose of OPV or IPV.
	Measles	All susceptible travelers born after 1957
	Rubella	Susceptible women of childbearing age
	Diphtheria	Susceptible hosts traveling to underdeveloped countries **(continued)**

Patient category	Vaccine	Comment
	Yellow fever & cholera	Countries requiring vaccination must have an international certificate of vaccination; offering locations available from state and local health departments
	Typhoid, plague, meningococcal disease, rabies, HBV or IG for HAV	Depends on risk in the country visited

*Td - Diphtheria and tetanus toxoids adsorbed (for adult use).

** Primary series in adults is three doses of Td toxoids with two doses given at least 4 weeks apart and a third dose given at 6-12 months after the second. Persons with unknown histories should be considered unvaccinated.

*** Persons are considered immune to measles and mumps if they have a dated record of vaccination with live virus vaccine on or before their first birthday, documented disease or laboratory evidence of immunity. Persons are considered immune to rubella if they have a record of vaccination by their first birthday or laboratory evidence of immunity. The preferred vaccine for persons susceptible to two or three is the combined measles, mumps, rubella (MMR) vaccine.

**** Live virus vaccines = Measles, rubella, yellow fever, oral polio vaccine (OPV).

Influenza Vaccine (Recommendations of the Advisory Committee on Immunization Practice: MMWR 36:373-387,1987; 37:361-373,1988; and 38:183-185,1989)

Preparations: Inactivated egg grown viruses that may be split (chemically treated to reduce febrile reactions in children) or whole. Preparations for the 1989-90 season contain 15 μg each of A/Taiwan/1/86 (H1N1), A/Shanghai/11/87-like antigen (H3N2) and B/Yamagata/16/88-like antigens/ 0.5 ml dose. Product information available from Connaught (800) 822-2463, Parke Davis (800) 223-0432 and Wyeth (800) 321-2304. A history of prior vaccination in any prior year does not preclude the need for revaccination. Remaining 1988-89 season vaccine should not be used.

Administration (over 12 years): Whole or split virus vaccine, 0.5 ml x 1 IM in the deltoid muscle, preferably in November and as early as September.

Target groups

1. Groups at greatest risk
   a. Adults and children with chronic disorders of the cardiovascular or pulmonary systems requiring regular medical following or hospitalization during the prior year.
   b. Residents of nursing homes or other chronic care facilities housing patients of any age with chronic medical conditions.

2. Groups at moderate risk
   a. Healthy individuals over 65 years.
   b. Persons who required regular medical following or hospitalization during prior year due to chronic metabolic disease (including diabetes mellitus, renal dysfunction, anemia or immunosuppression).
   c. Children (6 mo to 18 yrs) receiving long term aspirin treatment and therefore at risk for Reye's syndrome with influenza.

3. Persons capable of transmitting nosocomial influenza to high risk groups
   a. Physicians, nurses and other health care workers having extensive contact with high risk patients.
   b. Providers of care to high risk persons in the home setting, and household members.

4. Persons with HIV infection

5. Others: Any persons who wish to reduce chances of influenza, especially those providing essential community services, e.g. policemen, firemen, etc.

Contraindications

1. Severe allergy to eggs.
2. Persons with febrile illness (delay until symptoms abate).
3. Pregnancy is not viewed as a contraindication in women with high risk conditions, but it is preferred to vaccinate during the first trimester.

Rabies Vaccine Recommendation of Advisory Committee on Immunization Practice (MMWR 33:393-402,407-408,1984 and 37:217-218,1988)

Indications for post-exposure antirabies treatment

a. Type of exposure: Primarily bite; less frequently by saliva exposure to cuts, wounds of skin or mucous membranes; aerosol exposure is rare mechanism of transmission.

b. Animal species: Primarily carnivorous wild animals (especially raccoons, skunks, foxes and bats in the U.S.); dogs and cats are rarely infected in the U.S., but are common in some underdeveloped countries; rodents are rarely infected.

c. Circumstances of exposure: An unprovoked attack is most suspect.

Treatment

a. Unimmunized persons:
   Rabies immune globulin (RIG) 20 IU/kg with ½ dose infiltrated into wound site and remainder IM in the gluteal area plus human diploid cell rabies vaccine (HDVC) IM (deltoid) in five 1 ml doses on days 0,3,7,14 and 28.

b. Immunized persons (pre-exposure immunization with any rabies vaccine and history of documented antibody response):
   Two doses of HDVC IM (deltoid) in two 1 ml doses on day 0 and 3 and 28.

c. Pre-exposure vaccination: Three 1 ml doses HDVC IM in deltoid on days 0, 7, and 28.

d. Rabies Vaccine Adsorbed (RVA) is a new cell culture-derived rabies vaccine licensed 3/88 for pre and post-exposure prophylaxis. Timing of vaccinations is identical to that for HDCV: a) pre-exposure - three 1.0 mL doses IM in deltoid on days 0, 7, and 28; b) post-exposure - five 1.0 mL doses IM in deltoid on days 0, 3, 7, 14 and 28. RIG is given as described above.

Side effects of HDVC and RVA

Local reactions are common.

Mild reactions (headache, abdominal pain, nausea, dizziness, etc): 10-20%.

Allergic reactions (hives to anaphylaxis): 1/1000.

Hepatitis Vaccine (Recommendations of the Advisory Council on Immunization Practices: MMWR 34:313-335,1985; Ann Intern Med 107:353-357,1987; Friedman LS and Dienstag Disease-A-Month 32:314-385,1987; MMWR 37:342-351,1988, MMWR 36:354-360,1987)

A. Terms (MMWR 34:317,1985): See page 156

B. Vaccine recommendations

1. HAV: Immune globulin (IG)

		Dose	Frequency
a) Pre-exposure			
	Workers with non-human primates	0.06	q 4-6 mo.
	Travelers to developing countries		
	Visit less than 3 mo.	0.02	Once
	Visit over 3 mo.	0.02	q 4-6 mo.

b) Post-exposure (must be given within two weeks of exposure)

Close personal contacts and sexual partners

Day care centers: Staff and attendees when one case or at least two cases in families of attendees

Institutions for custodial care: Residents and staff with close contact with cases — 0.02 — Once

Common source exposure: food and waterborne outbreaks if recognized within the 2 week post-exposure period of effectiveness

Food handlers: Other food handlers, but not patrons unless uncooked food was handled without gloves and patrons can be located within 2 weeks of exposure

Hospitals: Not recommended for hospital personnel

2. Hepatitis B: (MMWR 36:353-366,1987; MMWR 37:342-351,1987)

a. Vaccine preparations
   (1) Heptavax B: Plasma-derived vaccine available since 6/82; 20 ug/ml.
   (2) Recombivax HB: Recombinant vaccine available since 7/86; 10 ug/ml.

b. Pre-exposure vaccination: Three IM doses (deltoid) at 0 time, 1 month and 6 months. The usual adult dose is 1 ml (20 ug plasma-derived or 10 ug of recombinant vaccine); immunosuppressed patients and hemodialysis patients should receive 40 ug doses of plasma-derived vaccine.

c. Screening to determine need for vaccine: Anti HBc or anti HBs (presence of these markers indicates protection and no need for vaccine).

Screening pregnant women: All pregnant women should be tested for HBsAg during an early prenatal visit; infants born to HBsAg positive mothers should receive HBIG (0.5 ml) IM x 1 (preferably within 12 hours of delivery) and HB vaccine (0.5 ml) x 3 (10 µg plasma derived or 5 µg recombinant) at 0 time (concurrent with HBIG), at 1 month and at 6 months. Test infant for HBsAg and anti-HBs at 12-15 mo.

d. Candidates for HBV vaccine:

Health care personnel exposed to blood and body fluids
Residents and staff of facilities for developmentally
    handicapped
Hemodialysis patients
IV drug abusers
Homosexual and bisexual men
Patients with hemoglobulinemias and clotting disorders
    requiring long term use of high risk plasma derivatives
Household and sexual contacts of HBV carriers
Miscellaneous groups for whom vaccine should be considered:
    inmates of long term correctional facilities; heterosexually active
    persons with multiple sexual partners; international travelers to
    HBV endemic areas

e. Post-exposure vaccination

(1) Percutaneous or needlestick injury

Source	Exposed person	
	Unvaccinated	Vaccinated
HBs Ag pos	HBIG* x 1 immediately Initiate HBV vaccine	Test for anti-HBs unless testing within past 12 mo. showed adequate Ab Positive: consider protected Negative: HBIG* immediately plus HBV vaccine booster
Known source High risk	Initiate HBV vaccine** Test source for HBsAg Positive: HBIG x 1	Test exposed for anti-HBs Positive: consider protected Negative: test source for HBsAg; if positive give HBIG* x 1 immediately plus HBV vaccine booster
Low risk	Initiate HBV vaccine series**	Nothing required
Unknown source	Initiate HBV vaccine series**	Nothing required

* HBIG = hepatitis immune globulin; usual dose is 0.06 ml/kg IM; it should be given as soon as possible after exposure and preferably within 24 hrs.
** HBV vaccine series refers to 3 doses at 0 time, 1 month, and 6 months; this should be initiated within 7 days of exposure; concurrent use with HBIG is acceptable, but separate IM injection sites should be used.

(2) Infants of HBsAg positive mothers (see 2c above).

f. Booster doses: Adults and children with normal immune status do not require serologic tests to assess antibody response and booster doses are not routinely recommended.

Hemodialysis patients: Test anti-HBs and give booster dose (20 μg plasma derived or 10 μg recombinant vaccine) if level is below 10 mIU/ml.

Pneumococcal Vaccine (Advisory Committee on Immunization Practices, Center For Disease Control, American Thoracic Society and Health and Public Policy Committee American College of Physicians: Ann Intern Med 101:348,1984; 104:118,1986; MMWR 38:64-76,1989)

<u>Vaccine:</u> 23 valent polysaccharide vaccine for the S. pneumoniae serotypes responsible for 87% of bacteremic pneumococcal disease in the U.S.

<u>Recommendations for adults</u>
1. Immunocompetent adults at increased risk of pneumococcal disease or its complications due to chronic illness (e.g. cardiovascular disease, pulmonary disease, diabetes, alcoholism, cirrhosis or cerebrospinal fluid leaks) or who are ≥65 years old.

2. Immunocompromised adults at increased risk of pneumococcal disease or its complications (e.g. splenic dysfunction or anatomic asplenia, lymphoma, Hodgkin's disease, multiple myeloma, nephrotic syndrome, alcoholism, renal failure and conditions associated with immunosuppression).

3. Adults with asymptomatic or symptomatic HIV infection.

Notations: 1) Vaccine should be given at least 2 weeks before elective splenectomy; 2) Vaccine should be given as long as possible before planned immunosuppressive treatment.

<u>Adverse reactions</u>
1. Pain and erythema at injection site: 50%
2. Fever, myalgia, severe local reaction: <1%
3. Anaphylactoid reactions: 5/million

<u>Revaccination:</u> Should be given once only. Arthus and other serological reactions are common in adults given second doses. Patients who received the 14 valent vaccine should not receive the 23 valent vaccine.

Tetanus Prophylaxis (MMWR 36:479,1987)

History of Tetanus toxoid	Clean, minor wounds		Other wounds**	
	Td*	TIG*	Td*	TIG*
Unknown or < 3 doses	Yes	No	Yes	Yes
≥ 3 doses	No, unless >10 yrs since last dose	No	No, unless 5 yrs since last dose	No

*Td = Tetanus toxoid; TIG = Tetanus immune globulin
** Wounds contaminated with dirt, stool, soil, saliva, etc; puncture wounds; avulsions; wounds from missiles, crushing, burns and frostbite.

Meningococcal Vaccine (Recommendation of Advisory Committee on Immunization Practices:MMWR 34:255,1985)

Preparation: Quadrivalent vaccine with immunogen (capsular polysaccharide) to serogroups A, C, Y and W-135. It lacks protection against serogroup B which accounts for 50-55% of cases in U.S.

Indications:

1) Outbreaks due to serogroups included in vaccine.
2) Persons with deficiencies of the terminal component of complement.
3) Persons with anatomic or functional asplenia.
4) Travelers to areas with hyperendemic or epidemic disease, especially those with prolonged contact with local populace. Representative area is the "meningitis belt" of sub-Saharan Africa (from Mauritania to Ethiopia).

Primary immunization: Single 0.5 ml dose

Revaccination: Indications unclear

PROPHYLACTIC ANTIBIOTICS

Antimicrobial Agents in Surgery (Adapted from the Medical Letter 29:91-94,1987 and Kaiser AB: New Engl J Med 315:1129-1138,1986)

Type of surgery	Preferred regimen	Alternative	Comment
CARDIOTHORACIC			
Cardiovascular: Coronary by-pass; valve surgery	Cefazolin 1 gm IV pre-op (and q6h x 48h)*	Vancomycin** 15 mg/kg IV pre-op, after initiation of by-pass (10 mg/kg) (and q8h x 48h)	Single doses appear to be as effective as multiple doses providing high serum concentrations are maintained throughout the procedure.
Pacemaker insertion	Cefazolin as above (see comments)	No alternative	Single doses appear to be as effective as multiple doses. Prophylaxis advocated only for centers with high infection rates.
Peripheral vascular surgery	Cefazolin 1 gm IV/IM pre-op (and q6h x 48h)*	Vancomycin** 15 mg/kg (and q8h x 48h)	Recommended for procedures on abdominal aorta and procedures on leg that include groin incision.
Thoracic surgery: lobectomy, pneumonectomy	Cefazolin 1 gm IV pre-op (and q6h x 48h)*		Optimal duration is unknown. Antibiotic prophylaxis is not recommended for thoracic trauma or chest tube insertion.

(continued)

69

Type of Surgery	Preferred regimen	Alternative	Comment
GASTROINTESTINAL			
Gastric surgery	Cefazolin 1 gm IV/IM pre-op	Clindamycin 600 mg IV + gentamicin 1.5 mg/kg	Advocated only for high risk - bleeding ulcer, obstruction, gastric ulcer, gastric cancer, gastric by-pass and percutaneous endoscopic gastrostomy. Prophylactic antibiotics are not indicated for uncomplicated duodenal ulcer surgery.
Biliary tract	Cefazolin 1 gm IV/IM pre-op	Gentamicin 1.5 mg/kg pre-op and q8h x 3	Advocated only for high risk - acute cholecystitis, obstructive jaundice, common duct stones, age over 70 yrs.
Colorectal	Neomycin 1 gm po and erythromycin 1 gm po at 1 pm, 2 pm and 11 pm the day before surgery (19,18 and 11 hrs pre-op)	Cefoxitin 1-2 gm IV or Clindamycin 600 mg IV plus gentamicin 1.5 mg/kg IV or Metronidazole 500 mg IV plus gentamicin 1.5 mg/kg IV	Some advocate the combined use of an oral and parenteral prep, especially for low anterior resection. Some advocate 3 subsequent doses of parenteral agents at 8 hr intervals.
Penetrating trauma abdomen	Cefoxitin 2 gm IV pre-op or Clindamycin 600 mg IV plus gentamicin 1.5 mg/kg pre-op		Patients with intestinal perforation should receive these agents for 2-5 days.

(continued)

Type of Surgery	Preferred regimen	Alternative	Comment
Appendectomy	Cefoxitin 1-2 gm IV pre-op (and 1-5 days post-op - see comments)	Metronidazole 500 mg (see comments)	For perforated or gangrenous appendix continue regimen for 3-5 days. For non-perforated appendix 1-4 doses are adequate.
Laparotomy, lysis of adhesions, splenectomy, etc. without GI tract surgery	None		

GYNECOLOGY AND OBSTETRICS

Type of Surgery	Preferred regimen	Alternative	Comment
Vaginal and abdominal hysterectomy	Cefazolin 1 gm IV/IM pre-op (and q6h x 2)*	Doxycycline 200 mg IV	Single dose appears to be as effective as multiple doses.
Cesarean section	Cefazolin 1 gm IV after clamping cord (and q6h x2)*	Metronidazole 500 mg IV or uterine irrigation with cefoxitin 2 gm in 1L normal saline	Advocated for high risk only - active labor, premature rupture of membranes
Abortion First trimester with PID	Aqueous penicillin G 1 million units IV pre-op.		Some advocate a second dose at 3 hrs post procedure.
Second trimester	Cefazolin 1 gm IV/IM pre-op	Metronidazole 500 mg po pre-op	Some advocate two additional doses.
Dilation and curettage	None		
Tubal ligation	None		
Cystocele or rectocele repair	None		

(continued)

Type of Surgery	Preferred regimen	Alternative	Comment
HEAD AND NECK			
Tonsillectomy ± adenoidectomy	None		
Rhinoplasty	None		
Major surgery with entry via oral cavity or pharynx	Cefazolin 1 gm IV/IM pre-op	Clindamycin 600 mg IV plus gentamicin 1.5 mg/kg IV pre-op and q8h x 2	
ORTHOPEDIC SURGERY			
Joint replacement	Cefazolin 1 gm IV/IM pre-op (and q6h x 3 doses)*	Vancomycin** 1 gm IV	Cefazolin dose should be 2 gm for knee replacement with tourniquet
Open reduction of fracture/internal fixation	Cefazolin 1 gm IV (and q6h x 3 doses)*		Open fractures are considered contaminated and should be treated with cefazolin 1 gm IV/IM q8h x 10 days*.
Amputation of leg	Cefoxitin 1-2 gm IV pre-op and q6h x 48h		
NEUROSURGERY			
Cerebrospinal fluid shunt	Trimethoprim 160 mg plus sulfamethoxazole 800 mg IV pre-op and q12h x 3 doses		Efficacy not clearly established
Craniotomy	Vancomycin 1 gm IV plus gentamicin 1.5 mg/kg	Clindamycin 300 mg IV and at 4 hr	Efficacy not clearly established. Advocated for pre-op high risk procedures - re-exploration and microsurgery.

Type of Surgery	Preferred regimen	Alternative	Comment
Spinal surgery	None		
UROLOGY			
Prostectomy			
Sterile urine	None		
Infected urine	Continue agent active in vitro		
Prostatic biopsy	None		
Dilation of urethra	None		
MISCELLANEOUS			
Inguinal hernia repair	None		
Mastectomy	None		

* Single dose generally considered adequate; for dirty surgery, treatment should be continued 5-10 days.

** Vancomycin preferred for hospitals with a high rate of wound infections caused by methicillin-resistant S. aureus or S. epidermidis, and for patients with allergy to penicillins or cephalosporins.

73

Prophylactic Antibiotics to Prevent Endocarditis in the Susceptible Host. Recommendations based on guidelines from the Committee on Prevention of Rheumatic Fever and Bacterial Endocarditis of the American Heart Association (Circulation 70:1123A–1127A,1984) and Medical Letter consultants (Medical Letter on Drugs and Therapeutics 29:107,1987)

A. **Patients to receive prophylaxis** (list is not considered all inclusive)

1. Valvular heart disease

   a. Prosthetic valve (including biosynthetic valves)

   b. Rheumatic valve disease (history of rheumatic fever without valve disease is not an indication)

   c. Congenital valve disease; an exception is uncomplicated atrial septal defect

   d. Prior history of endocarditis

2. Mitral valve prolapse if associated with a mitral insufficiency murmur

3. Idiopathic hypertrophic subaortic stenosis

4. Surgically constructed systemic-pulmonary shunts

B. **Procedures with established or suspected risk**

1. Respiratory tract

   a. All dental procedures likely to cause gingival bleeding

   b. Tonsillectomy and/or adenectomy

   c. Surgical procedures or biopsy of the respiratory mucosa

   d. Bronchoscopy, especially with a rigid bronchoscope (risk with flexible bronchoscope is low)

   e. Incision and drainage of infected tissue

2. Gastrointestinal and genitourinary tract

   a. Surgery or instrumentation of the genitourinary tract and gastrointestinal tract

      (1) Urology: Cystoscopy, prostatic surgery, urethral catheterization (especially with urinary tract infection), GU tract surgery

(2) Gastrointestinal tract: Esophageal dilatation, gallbladder surgery, scleral therapy of varices, colonic surgery.

(3) Endoscopy: Upper GI endoscopy with biopsy, proctosigmoidoscopy with biopsy

(4) Female genital tract: Obstetrical infections (but not for routine deliveries), and vaginal hysterectomy

b. Incision and drainage of infected tissue

c. Prophylaxis is not recommended for percutaneous liver biopsy, GI endoscopy without biopsy, barium enema, uncomplicated vaginal delivery, brief ("in and out") urinary catheterization with sterile urine, cesarean section, therapeutic abortions, uterine dilatation and curettage, sterilization procedures, insertion of IUD.

d. The risk appears enhanced for patients with prosthetic valves or surgically constructed systemic-pulmonary shunts. The Committee recommends only parenteral regimens and more liberal use of prophylaxis for these patients.

C. **Regimens** (Medical Letter 29:107,1985)

1. Procedures involving dental work and the respiratory tract

Pre-procedure	Subsequent doses
a. Parenteral	
(1) Ampicillin, 2 gm IM or IV 30 min pre-procedure plus gentamicin, 1.5 mg/kg IM or IV 30 min pre-procedure	Options: Repeat parenteral regimen 8 hrs later; give penicillin V, 1 gm po 8 hr later, or give no further antibiotics (Medical Letter consultants do not recommend the second dose)
(2) Penicillin allergy: Vancomycin, 1 gm IV starting 1 hr prior to procedure	None
b. Oral (not recommended for patients with prosthetic valves)	
(1) Penicillin V, 2 gm, po, 1 hr pre-procedure	Penicillin V, 1 gm po 6 hr later
(2) Penicillin allergy: Erythromycin, 1 gm po 1 hr pre-procedure	Erythromycin, 500 mg po 6 hr later

2. Procedures involving GI or GU tract

	Pre-procedure	Subsequent doses
a.	Parenteral	
	(1) Ampicillin, 2 gm IM or IV 30 min pre-procedure plus gentamicin, 1.5 mg/kg IM or IV 30 min pre-procedure	None
	(2) Penicillin allergy: Vancomycin, 1 gm infused over 1 hr beginning 1 hr pre-procedure plus gentamicin, 1.5 mg/kg IM or IV 30 min pre-procedure	None
b.	Oral (not recommended for patients with prosthetic valves, prior endocarditis or for patients receiving oral penicillin prophylaxis for rheumatic fever)	
	Amoxicillin, 3 gm po 1 hr pre-procedure	Amoxicillin, 1.5 gm po 6 hr later

TRAVELER'S DIARRHEA

(Adapted from NIH Consensus Development Panel,1985; see JAMA 253:2700,1985)

Risk: High risk areas (incidence 20-50%): developing countries of Latin America, Africa, Middle East and Asia.

Intermediate risk: Southern Europe and some Caribbean islands.

Low risk: Canada, Northern Europe, Australia, New Zealand, United States.

Agents

Bacteria
E. coli (enterotoxigenic,* enteroinvasive, enteroadherent)
Salmonella
Shigella
Campylobacter jejuni
Aeromonas hydrophila
Yersinia enterocolitica
Plesiomonas shigelloides
Vibrio cholerae (non-01)
Vibrio fluvialis
Vibrio parahaemolyticus

Viruses
Norwalk agent
Rotavirus (?)

Parasites
Giardia lamblia
Entamoeba histolytica
Cryptosporidium

* Most common

Prevention

Food and beverages: Risky foods - Raw vegetables, raw meat or raw seafood, tapwater, ice, unpasturized milk and dairy products and unpeeled fruit.

Preventative agents with documented efficacy (efficacy of 50-85%)
Doxycycline: 100 mg po/day
Sulfa-trimethoprim: 1 DS (double strength) tab po/day
Bismuth subsalicylate (Pepto-Bismol): 2 oz po qid or 2 300 mg tabs qid

Treatment

Oral intake to maintain fluid and electrolyte balance:
Potable fruit juice, caffeine-free soft drinks, salted crackers
For severe symptoms: WHO oral replacement solution that may be formulated by -

Ingredients/L or qt. water
NaCl: 3.5 gm (3/4 tsp)
NaHCO3 (baking soda): 2.5 gm (1 tsp)
KCl: 1.5 g (1 cup orange juice or 2 bananas)
Sucrose (table sugar): 40 gm (4 level tbsp)

Antimotility drugs
  Diphenoxylate (Lomotil) (2 2.5 mg tabs po 3-4 x daily)
  Loperamide (Imodium) (4 mg, then 2 mg after each loose stool to maximum
    of 16 mg/day)
  Bismuth subsalicylate (Pepto-Bismol) (30 ml or 2 tabs q 30 min x 8)

Antimicrobial agents (empiric selection)
  Sulfa-trimethoprim: 1 DS tab bid x 5 days
  Trimethoprim: 200 mg bid x 5 days
  Doxycycline: 100 mg bid x 5 days

Panel Recommendations

1. Prophylactic drugs are not recommended (but prophylactic antimicrobial
   agents appear most cost-effective; see Reves RR et al: Arch Intern Med
   148:2421,1988).

2. Travelers to risk areas should carry antimotility drugs (diphenoxylate or
   loperamide) or bismuth subsalicylate and an antimicrobial agent (sulfa-
   trimethoprim, trimethoprim or doxycycline).

   a. Mild diarrhea (less than 3 stools/day, without blood, pus or fever):
      Loperamide, dipenyoxylate or bismuth subsalicylate in doses noted above.

   b. Moderate or severe diarrhea: Antimicrobial agent (regimens noted above).

   c. Persistent diarrhea with serious fluid loss, fever or stools showing blood
      or mucus: Seek medical attention.

3. Instruct patients regarding
   Dietary precautions for prevention
   Oral rehydration
   Use of drugs including side effects

TREATMENT OF FUNGAL INFECTIONS
Adapted from NIAID Mycosis Study Group Reports (Ann Intern Med 98:13,1983; Ann Intern Med 103:861,1985; Chest 93:848,1987) and recommendations of the American Thoracic Society (Amer Rev Resp Dis 138:1078,1988)

Fungus	Form	Preferred treatment	Dose, alternative agent(s), comment
Aspergillus	Bronchopulmonary allergic	Corticosteroids	
	Aspergilloma (fungus ball)	Usually none	Massive hemoptysis-surgical resection with perioperative amphotericin. Progressive invasive disease - amphotericin B IV, 30-40 mg/kg
	Invasive pulmonary or or extrapulmonary	Amphotericin B IV	Total dose: 30-40 mg/kg Most patients require rapid advance in daily dose to 0.5-1.0 mg/kg Surgery often required for pulmonary cavities and sinus infections
Blastomyces	Acute pulmonary (immunocompetent)	Usually none	
	Acute pulmonary - severe or progressive	Ketoconazole po	400 mg/day; with unfavorable clinical response - increase to 600-800 mg/day Alternative: Amphotericin B IV, 30-40 mg/kg
	Chronic pulmonary	Ketoconazole po	As above **(continued)**

Fungus	Form	Preferred treatment	Dose, alternative agent(s), comment
	Disseminated (immunocompetent without renal or CNS involvement)	Ketoconazole po	As above
	Disseminated with GU involvement	Ketoconazole po	600–800 mg/day Alternative: Amphotericin B IV, 30–40 mg/kg
	Disseminated Immunosuppressed or CNS involvement	Amphotericin B IV	Total dose: 30–40 mg/kg
Candida	Localized-mucocutaneous		
	Oral (thrush)	Nystatin S&S Clotrimazole Ketoconazole	500,000 units 3-5x/day x 10-14d 10 mg troches 3-5x/day x 10-14d 200 mg po bid, 5-7 days AIDS: Continue any of above regimens indefinitely
	Vaginal	Miconazole Nystatin Clotrimazole Ketoconazole	Intravaginal cream (2%) or suppository (100 mg) qd x 7d Intravaginal cream or tablet (100,000 units) bid x 7d Intravaginal cream (1%) or tablet (100 mg) qd x 7d 200 mg po bid x 5-7d **(continued)**

Fungus	Form	Preferred treatment	Dose, alternative agent(s), comment
	Cutaneous - intertrigo balanitis, paronychia	Nystatin, ciclopirox, clotrimazole, miconazole	Topical treatment, keep area dry and clean with maximum exposure to air
	Chronic mucocutaneous	Ketoconazole	200 mg po bid x 3-12 months Alternative: Intermittent amphotericin B ± topical anti-Candida agent
	Esophageal	Ketoconazole	200 mg po bid x 10-14d Alternative: Amphotericin B (0.2-0.4 mg/kg/day) x 7-14 days AIDS: Maintenance ketoconazole 200 mg po bid
	Peritoneal (peritoneal dialysis)	Amphotericin B topical or IV	Topical treatment: 2-4 µg/L in dialysate fluid Catheter may require removal
	Peritoneal - (post-op, perforated viscus, etc)	Amphotericin B IV	Total dose: 3-10 mg/kg (Indications to treat are often unclear)
	Urinary	None or Amphotericin B topically	Remove catheter or use for bladder instillations of amphotericin B: 50 mg/L in D5W and infuse 1 L/day via closed triple lumen catheter x 5 days Alternative: Flucytosine Fungus ball: Surgical removal and amphotericin B IV **(continued)**

Fungus	Form	Preferred treatment	Dose, alternative agent(s), comment
	Bloodstream Septicemia	Amphotericin B IV	Total dose: 3-10 mg/kg Remove or change IV lines Immunocompetent host: Remove line and treat only if fungemia persists Immunosuppressed: Remove line, but treatment with amphotericin B ± flucytosine often required
	Disseminated or metastatic (deep organ infection)	Amphotericin B IV ± flucytosine po	Total dose: 20-40 mg/kg (0.3-0.8 mg/kg/day) Indications for flucytosine: Normal marrow and renal function or clinical deterioration with amphotericin B Flucytosine dose: 150 mg/kg/day po Alternative: Ketoconazole or miconazole for patients who refuse or cannot tolerate amphotericin B
	Endocarditis	Amphotericin B IV ± flucytosine po	Total dose: 30-40 mg/kg 150 mg/kg/day (flucytosine) Surgery required
Chromoblastomycosis		Fluconazole po	100-150 mg/kg/day x 6-8 wks Alternatives: Ketoconazole po 400 mg/day x 3-6 mo, thiabendazole or intra-lesional amphotericin B **(continued)**

Fungus	Form	Preferred treatment	Dose, alternative agent(s), comment
			Small lesions usually respond to fluconazole; large lesions should be surgically excised with perioperative fluconazole
Coccidioides	Pulmonary - acute	Usually none	
	Pulmonary - severe, cavitary or progressive infiltrate	Ketoconazole po or amphotericin B IV	400-600 mg/day x 6-18 mo. 15-40 mg/kg (amphotericin)
	Pulmonary cavitary disease - giant cavities (>5 cm, sub-pleural location, serious hemoptysis and secondary infection	Surgical excision	Perioperative amphotericin B often advocated (500 mg)
	Disseminated (non-meningeal, immunocompetent)	Amphotericin B IV or ketoconazole	Total dose: 30-40 mg/kg (amphotericin) Note: Relapses appear more common with ketoconazole Ketoconazole in dose of 200-800 mg/day (usually 400-600 mg) x 6-18 mo. or longer
	Disseminated - immunosuppressed non-meningeal	Amphotericin B IV	Total dose: 30-40 mg/kg
	Meningitis	Amphotericin B IV and topically	Total dose: 30-40 mg/kg IV Intrathecal: 0.5-0.7 mg 2x/wk Alternative: Miconazole or ketoconazole (800-1200 mg/day) (experience limited) **(continued)**

Fungus	Form	Preferred treatment	Dose, alternative agent(s), comment
Cryptococcus	Pulmonary-stable and immunocompetent	Usually none	Exclude extrapulmonary disease: culture blood, urine and CSF; follow x rays q 1-2 mo. x 1 yr
	Pulmonary - progressive and/or immunosuppressed host	Amphotericin B IV ± flucytosine	Total dose: 15-20 mg/kg (amphotericin) Alternative for immunocompetent host with progressive pulmonary or extrapulmonary non-meningeal is ketoconazole 200-800 mg po/day
	Extrapulmonary non-meningeal	Amphotericin B ± flucytosine	Total dose: 2-3 gm (amphotericin B) Alternative for immunocompetent patient is ketoconazole 400 mg/day
	Disseminated including meningeal	Amphotericin B ± flucytosine	Standard: Amphotericin (0.3 mg/kg/day) + flucytosine (150 mg/kg/day) x 6 weeks Four week regimen: Immuno-competent host without neurologic complications, pretreatment CSF WBC > 20/mm^3 + Ag < 1:32; and post therapy CSF Ag < 1:8 + neg India ink
			AIDS: Amphotericin B, 0.4-0.6 mg/kg/day ± flucytosine x 6-10 wks; then maintenance amphotericin B IV 1 mg/kg/wk, ketoconazole 400 mg po/day (non-meningeal only) or fluconazole (experimental) 200-400 mg po qd **(continued)**

Fungus	Form	Preferred treatment	Dose, alternative agent(s), comment
Histoplasma	Pulmonary - acute	Usually none	Severe acute: Some recommend amphotericin B (500 mg over 2-3 wks) or ketoconazole (400 mg/day) x 6 mo.
	Pulmonary - chronic	Amphotericin B	Total dose: 35-40 mg/kg Alternative: Ketoconazole, 400-600 mg/day x 6 mo. Relapses more common with ketoconazole
	Pulmonary - cavitary Stable, minimal sx, thin wall cavity	None	
	Persistent, thick walled cavity (> 2mm) or progressive sx	Ketoconazole po	400-800 mg/day x 6-12 mo. Alternative: Amphotericin B IV, 30-40 mg/kg Surgery for intractable hemoptysis despite medical Rx
	Disseminated - Immunocompetent, without CNS involvement	Ketoconazole po	As above
	Disseminated - CNS involvement or immunosuppressed	Amphotericin B IV	Total dose: 30-40 mg/kg AIDS: Amphotericin in dose of 0.5-1.0 gm, then maintenance ketoconazole po 400 mg/day or amphotericin B IV 1 mg/kg/wk **(continued)**

Fungus	Form	Preferred treatment	Dose, alternative agent(s), comment
	Mediastinal granuloma or fibrosis	Surgical resection if symptomatic	Invasive disease into airways, esophagus, etc (rare): Treat with ketoconazole or amphotericin B
	Ocular	Laser photocoagulation Intraocular steroids Retinal irradiation	Appears to be immune-mediated disease
Paracoccidioides	Pulmonary or mucocutaneous	Ketoconazole po	200-400 mg/day x 6-12 mo. Alternative: Amphotericin B IV, 30-40 mg/kg (preferred for severe disease) or sulfonamides
Phycomycetes Absidia Rhizopus Mucor (Mucormycosis)	Pulmonary and extrapulmonary including rhinocerebral	Amphotericin B IV	Total dose: 30-40 mg/kg Most patients require rapid increase to daily dose of 0.5-1.0 mg/kg Rhinocerebral: Surgical debridement required
Pseudoallescheria boydii	Sinusitis, endophthalmitis	Ketoconazole po or miconazole IV	200-600 mg/day x 1-12 mo 200-1200 mg q8h
Sporothrix (Sporotrichosis)	Lymphocutaneous	SSKI po	1 ml (1 gm/ml) tid increasing to 12-15 ml/day x 6-8 wks Alternative: Ketoconazole
	Extracutaneous	Amphotericin B IV	Total dose: 30-40 mg/kg

Antifungal Agents

Amphotericin B

A. <u>Activity</u>: Active *vs* most fungi including Aspergillus, Blastomyces, Candida (all species), Cryptococcus, Histoplasma, Coccidioides, Phycomycetes (Absidia, Rhizopus, Mucor), and Sporothrix. Resistance has been noted in strains of Coccioides, Candida, Pseudoallescheria and Phycomycetes

B. <u>Administration</u>

1. IV administration: Dissolve in D5W in concentration less than 0.1 mg/ml and deliver by slow infusion over 4-6 hrs with or without
   1) heparin (50 units/dl in the infusion) to reduce phlebitis,
   2) hydrocortisone (25-50 mg IV) to reduce fever and chills,
   3) premedication with ASA (15-20 mg/kg po), diphenhydramine (Benadryl 25 mg po) and meperidine HCl (15-20 mg IV)

   a. Initial dose: 1 mg in 50-100 mL D5W infused IV over 20 hrs with monitoring over 4 hrs of vital signs to detect hypersensitivity reaction, hypotension, etc. (Some simply start with a 5-10 mg dose)

   b. Standard regimen: .25 mg/kg in 500 ml D5W over 2-6 hrs; with subsequent dose increases of 5-10 mg/day to maintenance doses.

   c. "Rapid regimen": Follow initial dose by 0.3 mg/kg at 4 hrs after test dose and then 2-3 doses at 8 hr intervals, but no more than 0.6 mg/kg/day.

   d. Maintenance: Usual dose is 0.3-0.7 mg/kg/day or 0.6-1.2 mg/kg qod given over 2-6 hours depending on tolerance; Maintenance doses for serious infections (Mucor, invasive aspergillosis) may be .8-1.2 mg/kg/day; the dose for less serious infections (candida esophagitis) is 0.3 mg/kg/day. Doses should be reduced or interval extended when serum creatinine exceeds 2.5 μg/dl. Usual total dose for deep seated mycotic infection is 1.5-3 gm; "Low dose maintenance regimen" is 0.3 mg/kg/day x 10 days.

   e. Monitoring during treatment: Serum creatinine daily or every other day; serum potassium, magnesium, and complete blood count 1-2x/week.

2. Local administration

   a. Intrathecal or intraventricular: Dissolve in D5W to give 0.25 mg/ml; 1st dose is 0.05 mg (50 μg) followed by 0.2-0.5 mg 1-3x weekly. Addition of dexamethasone 0.25 mg/ml may reduce local toxic effect. Volume of CSF equal to volume injected should be withdrawn before intrathecal administration. Usual method of administration is intraventricular via Ommaya reservoir.

b. Intravesicular: Continuous irrigation via triple lumen catheter using 50 mg/L D5W/day.

c. Intra-articular: 5-15 mg infusions.

d. Intra-ocular: Up to 10 μg.

C. Pharmacokinetic properties: Poor absorption with topical therapy (oral, bladder, joint instillations, etc). Peak serum levels are 1-3 μg/ml with usual dose (1 mg/kg 3x/wk). Stored in body and slowly released so that after discontinuation therapeutic serum levels are detectable up to 9 days, urinary excretion continues 2-4 months and tissue levels are detected for 1 yr. Serum half life is 24-48 hrs. Only 3-5% is excreted in urine so that renal failure has minimal effect on dosing recommendations. Penetration into the eye and CNS are poor. Due to unusual pharmacokinetic properties this is one of the few antimicrobial agents in which the recommended treatment strategies are given in terms of total dose rather than daily dose.

D. Side effects:

a. Chills, fever, headache, nausea, and vomiting; 50% of patients; reduce with slow infusion and aspirin, corticosteroids, antiemetics, IV meperidine, etc. Tolerance usually improves with continued treatment.

b. Nephrotoxicity: Early nephrotoxicity is reversible and dose related; late more irreversible damage is due to total dose. When renal function normal at start the incidence of residual renal disease with 2 gm is low and with over 4 gm it is expected. Usual manifestations are increasing creatinine, K loss, proteinuria and renal tubular acidosis.

c. Phlebitis at infusion site; reduce with concurrent heparin slow infusion or central line.

d. Anemia due to suppression of erythropoiesis; dose related and reversible. Leukopenia and thrombocytopenia also common.

e. Hypokalemia: K supplementation with alkalinizing salt (bicarbonate, gluconate, etc) often necessary.

f. Drug interaction with granulocytic transfusions (pulmonary infiltrates).

Flucytosine

A. Activity: Active vs. most strains of Phialophora, Cladosporium, Candida and Cryptococcus; activity vs. Aspergillus is variable.

B. Indications: Chromomycosis (caused by Phialophora and Cladosporium) is the only indication for flucytosine alone; usually used in combination with amphotericin.

C. Administration: 25-40 mg/kg (usually 37.5 mg/kg) po q6h; dosing interval is extended in renal failure:
Creatinine clearance > 40 ml/min - usual dose q6h.
Creatinine clearance 20-40 ml/min - usual dose q12h.
Creatinine clearance 10-20 ml/min - usual dose q24h.
Creatinine clearance <10 - maintain level 100 mg/ml
Peritoneal dialysis: usual dose q24h
Hemodialysis: usual dose post dialysis

D. Pharmacokinetics: Absorption 80-90% with oral dosing, usual peak serum level = 50-75 μg/ml; widely distributed with good penetration to eye and CNS. 90% eliminated unchanged in urine; half life of 3-5 hr increases to 100 hr in renal failure.

E. Side effects: Avoid or use with extreme caution in patients with renal failure (especially with concurrent amphotericin B) or marrow suppression (cancer chemotherapy, AIDS, AZT therapy, etc).

1. Nausea and/or diarrhea (6%); fatal enterocolitis with diarrhea and cramps reported.

2. Leukopenia and thrombocytopenia: Dose related, especially with levels over 100 mg/ml; concurrent cytosine arabinoside contraindicated. Monitoring serum levels is advocated, especially if given with renal failure or with nephrotoxic or marrow toxic drugs.

3. Hepatic dysfunction in 5-10%, reversible.

4. Teratogenic: Contraindicated in pregnancy.

5. When combined with amphotericin B, there may be toxic blood levels due to the renal toxicity of amphotericin.

Ketoconazole (Nizoral)

A. Activity: Candida sp, Blastomyces, Coccidioides, Histoplasma, Paracoccidioides, Cryptococcus, Pseudoallescheria boydii and dermatophytes.

B. Administration: 200 mg tablets; usual dose is 200-400 mg/day, but doses up to 800-1,200 mg/day have been given for 6 months or longer depending on infection (see treatment of fungal infections). Drug is well absorbed only in persons with normal gastric acidity so achlorhydria or concurrent use of antacids or H2-blocking agents interferes with absorption; patients with achlorhydria should swallow the drug as one 200 mg tab dissolved in 4 ml of 0.2 N HCl and those requiring antacids, H2 blockers or anti-cholinergics should receive them at least 2 hours after ketoconazole. Dose should be reduced in liver disease, but specific guidelines are not available.

C. Pharmacokinetics: Mean peak serum levels with 200 and 400 mg doses are 2 and 4 ug/ml, respectively. Penetrates into body fluids and tissues well except CNS. Serum half life is 1.5-9 hours depending on dose and is not altered by renal failure. Metabolized in the liver and inactive metabolites are excreted in the bile; urine levels are nil.

D. Side effects:

1. Gastrointestinal: Nausea, vomiting, anorexia are common and dose dependent.

2. Inhibition of testosterone synthesis with impotence, decreased libido, gynecomastia; dose related.

3. Interferes with cortisol synthesis although hypodrenalism is rare.

4. Hepatic toxicity with increased aminotransferase levels is common (2-10%) and usually reversible with continued use; 1 in 15,000 develops symptomatic hepatitis that may be fatal and is not dose related. The patient should report any symptoms of liver disease such as unusual fatigue, nausea, vomiting, jaundice, dark urine, or pale stools. It is recommended that liver function tests be examined before and at 1-2 month intervals during treatment.

5. Miscellaneous: Menstrual irregularities, pruritis, rash, headache, fever, dizziness, diarrhea, constipation.

6. Interactions: Avoid concurrent use of antacids, H2 blocking agents, anticholinergics, antiparkinsonism drugs, rifampin, isoniazide and phenytoin.

TREATMENT OF VIRAL INFECTIONS

A. Herpesvirus Group

Virus	Regimen	Comment
Herpes simplex		
Genital-primary	Acyclovir: Topical - q4h while awake x 7 days; oral - 200 mg 5 x daily x 5-10 days; IV 5-15 mg/kg/day x 5-7 days	Oral or intravenous therapy usually preferred Mild lesions and symptoms are usually not treated
Genital-recurrent	Acyclovir: Oral - 200 mg 5 x daily x 5-7 days	Initiate during prodrome or at first site of lesions
Genital-prophylaxis	Acyclovir: 200 mg 2-5 x/day up to 18 months	For patients with severe or frequent recurrences
Orolabial-immuncompetent host	None	
Encephalitis	Acyclovir: IV - 10 mg/kg q 8 h x 10-14 days	
Mucocutaneous progressive	Acyclovir: IV - 5-10 mg/kg q 8 h x 7-14 days; oral - 200-400 mg po 5 x/day x 7-14 days	AIDS patients often require preventative therapy with acyclovir 200-400 mg po tid indefinitely
Burn wound	Acyclovir: IV - 5 mg/kg q 8 h x 7 days; oral - 200 mg 5 x/day x 7-14 days	
Prophylaxis - high risk patients	Acyclovir: IV - 5 mg/kg q 8 h; oral - 400 mg 3-5 x/day	Organ transplant recipients (renal and marrow): treat seropositive patients for 1-3 mo. post transplant
Keratitis	Trifluorothymidine: Topical (1%) or Vidarabine: topical (3%) x 7-21 days	
Acyclovir - resistant strains	Vidarabine: IV 10-15 mg/kg over 12-24 hr Foscarnate: IV 60 mg/kg q8h (investigational)	Thymidine kinase deficient strains, usually in HSV-2 strains treated with acyclovir

91

Virus	Regimen	Comment
Varicella-zoster		
Immunocompetent		
Pneumonia	Acyclovir: IV 10-12 mg/kg q 8 h x 7 days; oral 800 mg 5 x daily x 10 days	Efficacy not established; IV preferred for serious infections due to relative resistance (compared to HSV) and poor oral absorption
Dermatomal	Acyclovir: IV 5 mg/kg or 250 mg/m^2 q 8 h x 5-7 days; oral 800 mg 5 x daily x 7-10 days	Efficacy of oral acyclovir for VZ is not established, but if used, large doses are advocated, eg. 800 mg 5 x/day
Ophthalmic zoster	Acyclovir: Oral 800 mg 5 x daily x 10 days	Consult ophthalmologist
Immunosuppressed		
Dermatomal zoster	Acyclovir: IV 10-12 mg/kg or 500 mg/m^2 q 8 h x 7 days	Alternative is vidarabine: 10 mg/kg/day IV x 5-7 days
Disseminated zoster or varicella	Acyclovir: IV 10-12 mg/kg or 500 mg/m^2 q 8 h x 7 days	Alternative is vidarabine: 10 mg/kg/day IV x 5-7 days
Cytomegalovirus		
Immunocompetent	None	
Immunosuppressed		
Retinitis	Ganciclovir (investigational) 5 mg/kg IV bid x 10-14 days	Efficacy established; maintenance therapy usually required using ganciclovir, 5 mg/kg/day IV
Colitis, enteritis, and esophagitis	Ganciclovir (investigational) 5 mg/kg IV bid x 10-14 days	Efficacy probable
Pneumonitis	Ganciclovir (investigational) 5 mg/kg IV bid x 10-14 days	Efficacy not established

Virus	Regimen	Comment
Prophylaxis: Renal transplant (see comment)	CMV immune globulin (investigational) 150 mg/kg within 72 hr, then 100 mg/kg at 2,4,6 & 8 wks, then 50 mg/kg at 12 & 16 wks	Indicated for CMV seronegative renal transplant recipient and CMV seronegative donors

B. Influenza A: Amantadine

A. Recommendations (Advisory Council on Immunization Practices: MMWR 37:361,1988)

1. Prophylaxis

Highest priority - Control presumed influenza A outbreaks in institutions with high risk persons; administer to all residents regardless of vaccination status as soon as possible after outbreak recognized and as long as there is influenza activity in community.

Other recommendations - **1)** As adjunct to late vaccination of high risk persons (two weeks required for vaccine response); **2)** Home care providers to reduce spread of infection and maintain care of high risk persons in home; **3)** Immunodeficient persons as supplement to vaccine, especially children with AIDS; **4)** Persons with contraindications to influenza vaccine.

2. Treatment: High risk patients with suspected influenza A; should be given within 24-48 hours after onset and continued until 48 hours after symptoms and signs resolve.

B. Dose (MMWR 37:373,1988)

1. Prophylaxis: 100 mg/day (all adults)

2. Treatment: Age 10-64 yrs - 200 mg/day in one or two doses
   Age > 65 yrs - 100 mg/day as single dose
   Seizure disorder - 100 mg/day

3. Creatinine clearance in ml/min/1.73 M^2(use ½ dose when 100 mg/day indicated)

   > 80: 200 mg/day
   60-80: 200 mg alternating with 100 mg/day
   40-60: 100 mg/day
   30-40: 200 mg twice weekly
   20-30: 100 mg three times weekly
   10-20: 200 mg alternating with 100 mg weekly

C. Side effects (dose related): Anxiety, insomnia, dizziness, drunk feeling, slurred speech, ataxia, depression, lightheadedness, inability to concentrate. Incidence is 5-10% for healthy young adults taking 200 mg/day; lower prophylactic dose presumably decreases side effects and retains efficacy.

C. AZT (Retrovir, Zidovudine)

__Indication:__ AIDS, ARC or HIV infection and CD4 count 500/mm^3

__Usual dose:__ 100-200 po q 4 h (5-6 x/day)

1. Asymptomatic with CD4 count ≤ 500/mm^3: 100 mg 5 x daily (q 4 h while awake)
2. AIDS or ARC with CD4 count < 200/mm^3: 200 mg 5-6 x daily (q 4 h or q 4 h while awake)
   a) Hepatic failure (ascites, jaundice, acute hepatitis): 200 mg po q 6 h*
   b) Renal failure (creatinine > 2 mg/dl): 200 mg q 6 h*

__Contraindications:__ Pretreatment Hgb<7 gm/dl or neutrophil count < 500/mm^3

Dose adjustment

Toxicity	Options
Hgb 6.5-7.9 gm/dl	Transfuse and/or dose reduction** until > 9.5 gm/dl or entry level; discontinue if transfusion requirement exceeds 2-3 units/2 weeks
< 6.5	Transfuse and discontinue** until > 9.5 gm/dl or entry level
WBC 1000-1500/mm^3	Dose reduction**
< 1000	Discontinue** until 2600/mm^3 or entry level
Granulocytes 500-750/mm^3	Dose reduction** until > 1300/mm^3 or entry level
< 500/mm^3	Discontinue** until > 1300/mm^3 or entry level
Platelets 25,000-50,000/mm^3	Dose reduction** until > 75,000/mm^3 or entry level
< 25,000	Discontinue** until > 75,000/mm^3 or entry level

* There are no clear guidelines for dose adjustment for renal failure, hepatic failure or small size thus, frequent hematologic monitoring is warranted.
** Dose reduction may be reduction to half dose or temporary discontinuation of the drug. When discontinued and restarted, use half dose. When counts improve dose may be escalated.

Toxicity

__Hematologic:__ Related to pretreatment marrow reserve, dose and duration.
   __a)__ Macrocytic anemia - as early as 2-4 wks; usually gradual.
   __b)__ Neutropenia - usually after 6-8 wks.
__Gastrointestinal:__ Nausea, vomiting, anorexia.
__CNS:__ Headache, somnolence, dizziness, insomnia; rare - confusion, cerebellar ataxia, stupor, seizures, myopathy with CPK elevation
__Miscellaneous:__ Fever, rash, nail pigmentation
__Rare:__ Anaphylaxis

Monitoring
1. CBC q 2-4 weeks.
2. Hepatic function q 4 weeks.

Drug interactions
Agents that affect hepatic glucuronidation: aspirin, cimetidine, indomethacin.
Agents that are nephrotoxic, cytotoxic or myelosuppressive: pentamidine, dapsone, amphotericin B, flucytosine, interferon, ganciclovir.
Probenecid: Prolongs half-life.   95

TREATMENT OF TUBERCULOSIS

Official statement of the American Thoracic Society and the Centers for Disease Control (Amer Rev Resp Dis 134:355-363,1986; 136:492-496,1987)

A. Initial treatment regimens (ATS and CDC recommendations)

1. Six month regimen
   Initial phase: INH, rifampin plus pyrazinamide given daily for 2 months (augment with ethambutol when INH resistance is suspected).

   Second phase: INH plus rifampin given daily or twice weekly for 4 months.

2. Nine month regimen
   INH plus rifampin for 9 months (augment with ethambutol when INH resistance is suspected; INH and rifampin should be given daily for 1-2 months and then daily or twice weekly).

3. Special considerations: Extrapulmonary tuberculosis, pregnancy, lactation, treatment failure, resistant strains, relapse and HIV infection: See F. Special Considerations (pg 98,99).

B. Recommended first line drugs

C. Second line antituberculous drugs (see next page)

Agent	Forms	Daily dose (maximum)	Adverse reactions	Monitoring
Capreomycin	Vials: 1 gm	15-30 mg/kg IM (1 gm)*	Auditory, vestibular and renal toxicity	Audiometry, vestibular function, renal function
Kanamycin	Vials: 75 mg, 500 mg and 1 gm	13-30 mg/kg IM (1 gm)*	Auditory, vestibular (rare), and renal toxicity	Audiometry, vestibular function, renal failure
Ethionamide	Tabs: 250 mg	15-20 mg/kg PO (1 gm)*	Gastrointestinal intolerance, hepatotoxicity, hypersensitivity	Hepatic enzymes
PAS	Tabs: 500 mg 1 gm	12 gm	Gastrointestinal intolerance, hepatotoxicity, sodium load, hypersensitivity	
Cycloserine	Caps: 250 mg	1 gm	Psychosis, rash, convulsions	Assess mental status

* Usual daily dose of adult

B. Recommended first line agents
(Amer Rev Resp Dis 134:355-363,1986 and Medical Letter 30:43,1988)

Agent	Forms	Daily dose (maximum)	Twice weekly dose (maximum)	Cost/mo. (daily regimen)	Adverse reactions	Comment
Isoniazid	Tabs: 100 mg, 300 mg Syrup: 50 mg/ 5 ml Vials: 1 gm	5 mg/kg po or IM (300 mg)*	15 mg/kg (900 mg)*	$1	Elevated hepatic enzymes, peripheral neuropathy, hepatitis, hypersensitivity	Oral or parenteral pyridoxine 15-50 mg/day to prevent neuropathy
Rifampin	Caps: 150 mg, 300 mg	10-20 mg/kg po (600 mg)*	10 mg/kg (600 mg)*	$13-21	Orange discoloration of secretions & urine, nausea, vomiting, hepatitis, fever, purpura (rare)	May be given as 10 mg/ml suspension
Pyrazinamide	Tabs: 500 mg	15-30 mg/kg po (2 gm)*	50-70 mg/kg	$19-48	Hepatotoxicity, hyperuricemia, arthralgias, rash, GI intolerance	
Streptomycin	Vials: 1 gm, 4 gm	15 mg/kg IM (1 gm)* pts> 40 yrs: 10 mg/kg IM (500-750 mg)*	25-30 mg/kg pts> 40 yrs: 20 mg/kg	$23-27	Ototoxicity and possible nephro-toxicity	Decrease dose for renal failure
Ethambutol	Tabs: 100 mg, 400 mg	15-25 mg/kg po (2.5 gm)*	50 mg/kg	$27-72	Optic neuritis, skin rash	25 mg/kg/day 1st 1-2 months or if strain is INH resistant. Decrease dose for renal failure

* Usual daily dose for adults.

D. **Monitoring for adverse reactions**

1. Baseline tests: Hepatic enzymes, bilirubin, serum creatinine or BUN, CBC, platelet count or estimate.
Pyrazinamide: uric acid; ethambutol: visual acuity.

2. During treatment: Clinical monitoring with assessment at least once monthly; laboratory monitoring is not recommended except for symptoms suggesting toxicity and in patients with pre-existing liver disease. (Hepatotoxicity from antituberculous drugs is not known to be more common in patients with prior liver disease).

E. **Evaluation of response**

1. Sputum examination (smear and culture): Monthly until conversion is documented; minimum is exam at 3 months: Review compliance and drug susceptibility.
Positive sputum at 3 months:

   a. Resistant organisms: Change regimen to include at least two active drugs and evaluate sputum susceptibility.

   b. Susceptible organisms: Review compliance.

2. Radiologic studies: At completion of treatment as baseline for comparison for future films; x-ray at 2-3 months of treatment may be useful.

3. Routine follow-up after treatment (sensitive organisms)
Nine month regimen with good response: None
Six month regimen: Follow-up at 6 and 12 months

F. **Special considerations**

1. Extrapulmonary tuberculosis

   a. Nine month two-drug regimen recommended for sensitive strains; consider longer treatment for lymphadenitis, bone and joint tuberculosis.

   b. Six month regimen is "probably effective".

   c. Some authorities recommend corticosteroids for tuberculosis pericarditis and meningitis.

2. Pregnancy and lactation

   a. INH plus rifampin; ethambutol should be added for suspected resistant strains.

   b. Streptomycin is only antituberculous drug with established fetal toxicity (interferes with ear development and causes congenital deafness); kanamycin and capreomycin presumably share this toxic potential.

   c. Breast feeding should not be discouraged.

98

3. Treatment failures (persistent positive cultures after 5-6 months)

   a. Susceptibility tests on current isolate while continuing same regimen or augmenting this with two additional drugs.

   b. Sensitive strain: Consider treatment under direct observation
      Resistant strain: Two active drugs
      INH resistance: Rifampin and ethambutol ± pyrazidamide for 12 months.

4. Relapse after treatment

   a. INH + rifampin regimen previously: Organism at time of relapse is usually sensitive if the original strain was. Therefore: Give same regimen initially, measure susceptibility, modify the regimen accordingly and consider observed treatment.

   b. Regimen not containing INH and rifampin: Presume new isolate is resistant to agents used. See 3b above.

5. HIV infection (Recommendations of the Centers for Disease Control and The American Thoracic Society: Amer Rev Resp Dis 136:492,1987)

   a. All patients with tuberculosis should have HIV serology.

   b. Antituberculous treatment should be started when acid-fast bacilli are are found in a patient with HIV infection pending cultures.

   c. Standard treatment (pulmonary TB)
      (1) Initial 2 mo: INH (300 mg/day), rifampin (600 mg/day or 450 mg/ day for patients < 50 kg) + pyrazinamide (20-30 mg/kg/day)
      (2) Duration: INH + rifampin to complete minimum of 9 months or at least 6 months after documented culture conversion; some authorities advocate continuing INH for lifetime.

   d. Disseminated disease, CNS involvement or suspected resistance: Add ethambutol (25 mg/kg/day) for initial treatment.

   e. Inability to include INH or rifampin: Treat for minimum of 18 months and for at least 12 months after documented culture conversion.

G. Preventative treatment

   1. Candidates for INH prophylaxis

      a. Household members and other close associates:

         (1) PPD skin reaction of 5 mm or more and no prior positive reaction - treat.

         (2) Patients with negative PPD and high risk (primarily children and adolescents) should be treated 3 months and then repeat PPD; if positive - complete course, if negative - discontinue INH.

99

b. Newly infected persons: Positive PPD with conversion within 2 years.

c. Persons with prior TB who have not received adequate treatment.

d. Persons with positive PPD and chest x-ray compatible with TB plus no evidence of active disease (negative cultures and stable parenchymal lesions).

e. Positive PPD in high risk groups:

(1) Silicosis.

(2) Diabetes mellitus, especially poorly controlled insulin-dependent patients.

(3) Corticosteroid therapy if dosage is over the equivalent of 15 mg/day prednisone for over 2-3 weeks. Treatment for those with low dose or alternative day dosing is controversial.

(4) Immunosuppressive therapy.

(5) AIDS or HIV infection with prior history of positive PPD (these patients may be anergic).

(6) Some hematologic and reticuloendothelial diseases such as leukemia and Hodgkin's disease.

(7) End stage renal disease with history of positive PPD (many patients are anergic).

(8) Conditions associated with rapid weight loss or chronic malnutrition including intestinal by-pass surgery, postgastrectomy state (with or without weight loss), chronic peptic ulcer disease, chronic malabsorption, carcinoma of the oropharynx or upper GI tract with inadequate nutrition.

f. Positive PPD in patient under 35 years.

2. Screening

a. Exclude active disease.

b. Exclude those with prior adequate course of INH.

c. Contraindications:

(1) Prior hepatitis or severe adverse reactions attributed to INH.

(2) Acute or active liver disease. Positive HBsAg is not a contraindication unless accompanied by acute or chronic hepatitis.

d. Assess relative risks: Age > 35 years, concurrent use of drugs that may cause interaction, daily use of alcohol, possible concurrent liver disease, or peripheral neuropathy or condition causing it (diabetes, alcoholism).

e. Pregnancy: Delay treatment until after delivery unless patient recently infected, when treatment is begun after first trimester.

f. HIV infection

   (1) Screening: Skin test (5 TU tuberculin); if patient has AIDS or HIV-related disease: skin test + chest x-ray and exam for extrapulmonary TB due to concern for false-negative skin tests with immunosuppression.

   (2) Preventative treatment in patients with positive skin tests: INH (300 mg/day) for 12 months regardless of age.

3. Regimen

   a. INH 300 mg/dag for 6-12 months (6 months confers nearly comparable protection, although patients with stable x-ray lesions and those with HIV infection should be treated 12 months).

   b. Alternative treatments:

      (1) Index case with INH resistant strain: (a) give INH, (b) give rifampin or rifampin plus ethambutol (for highly susceptible - child - or immunosuppressed host), or (c) observe.

      (2) Suspected INH resistance: Consider rifampin or observe.

      (3) INH intolerance: Consider rifampin or observe.

      (4) BCG vaccine: Consider only in PPD negative persons where INH cannot be used and there is continuing exposure to sputum-positive index case.

4. Monitoring

   a. Dispense in monthly allotments and patients should be queried at monthly intervals (by telephone or visit) regarding symptoms of hepatitis or other adverse reactions.

   b. Liver function tests should be obtained in patients with symptoms suggesting liver disease. Transaminase levels are recommended pre-treatment and periodically during treatment for patients over 35 years.

101

Atypical Mycobacteria

Agent	Condition	Treatment
M. kansasii	Major: Pulmonary	3 drugs x 18 mo.: INH, rifampin, and ethambutol Alternatives: Sulfamethoxazole, streptomycin
M. avium-intracellulare	Infrequent: Lymphadenopathy; disseminated disease	3-5 drugs x 2 yrs: INH, rifampin, ethambutol, pyrazinamide, streptomycin, ethionamide
	Immunocompetent: Pulmonary	3-5 drugs x 2 yrs: INH, rifampin, ethambutol, pyrazinamide, streptomycin, ethionamide
	AIDS: Disseminated disease	Efficacy of treatment debated; consider 3-5 drugs (above) plus ansamycin (in place of rifampin), clofazimine and/or amikacin
M. marium	Skin	Rifampin + ethambutol or trimethoprim-sulfa x 6 wks. Excision of lesions
M. ulcerans	Skin	Rifampin + amikacin, trimethoprim-sulfa or ethambutol x 4-6 wks Excision of lesions
M. fortuitum & M. chelonei	Post-operative sites (especially augmentation mammoplasty and median sternotomy); pulmonary; skin; lymphadenopathy; bone; keratitis	Cefoxitin + amikacin IV, then sulfonamide, rifampin, doxycycline or erythromycin orally (select by sensitivity tests) M. chelonae ss abscessus is usually sensitive to amikacin, cefoxitin and erythromycin; M. chelonei ss chelonae is usually sensitive to amikacin, tobramycin, erythromycin and doxycycline. Excision of lesions including removal of associated devices Ciprofloxacin is active vs M. fortuitum, but role in treatment is unknown.
M. gordonae	Pulmonary	INH, rifampin + ethambutol

TREATMENT OF PARASITIC INFECTIONS
(Reprinted from The Medical Letter on Drugs and Therapeutics 30:16,1988, with permission)

Infection	Drug	Adult Dosage*
AMEBIASIS (Entamoeba histolytica)		
asymptomatic		
Drug of choice:	Iodoquinol[1]	650 mg tid x 20d
Alternatives:	Diloxanide furoate[2]	500 mg tid x 10d
	Paromomycin	25-30 mg/kg/d in 3 doses x 7d
mild to moderate intestinal disease		
Drugs of choice:	Metronidazole[3,4]	750 mg tid x 10d
	followed by iodo-quinol[1]	650 mg tid x 20d
Alternative:	Paromomycin	25-30 mg/kg/d in 3 doses x 7d
severe intestinal disease		
Drugs of choice:	Metronidazole[3,4]	750 mg tid x 10d
	followed by iodo-quinol[1]	650 mg tid x 20d
Alternatives:	Dehydroemetine[2,5]	1 to 1.5 mg/kg/d (max. 90 mg/d) IM for up to 5d
	followed by iodo-quinol[1]	650 mg tid x 20d
	OR Emetine[5]	1 mg/kg/d (max. 60 mg/d) IM for up to 5d
	followed by iodo-quinol[1]	650 mg tid x 20d
hepatic abscess		
Drugs of choice:	Metronidazole[3,4]	750 mg tid x 10d
	followed by iodo-quinol[1]	650 mg tid x 20d
Alternatives:	Dehydroemetine[2,5]	1 to 1.5 mg/kg/d (max. 90 mg/d) IM for up to 5d
	followed by chloroquine phos-phate	600 mg base (1 gram)/d x 2d, then 300 mg base (500 mg)/d x 2-3 wks
	plus iodoquinol[1]	650 mg tid x 20d
	OR Emetine[5]	1 mg/kg/d (max. 60 mg/d) IM for up to 5d
	followed by chloroquine phos-phate	600 mg base (1 gram)/d x 2d, then 300 mg base (500 mg)/d x 2-3 wks
	plus iodoquinol[1]	650 mg tid x 20d
AMEBIC MENINGOENCEPHALITIS, PRIMARY		
Naegleria sp		
Drug of choice:	Amphotericin B[6,7]	1 mg/kg/d IV, uncertain duration
Acanthamoeba sp		
Drug of choice:	see footnote 8	
Ancylostoma duodenale, see HOOKWORM		
ANGIOSTRONGYLIASIS		
Angiostrongylus cantonensis		
Drug of choice:	Mebendazole[7,9,10]	100 mg bid x 5d
Angiostrongylus costaricensis		
Drug of choice:	Thiabendazole[7,9]	25 mg/kg tid x 3d[11] (max. 3 grams/day)
	OR surgical intervention	
ANISAKIASIS (Anisakis sp)		
Treatment of choice:	Surgical removal	

103

Infection	Drug	Adult Dosage*
ASCARIASIS (Ascaris lumbricoides, roundworm)		
Drug of choice:	Mebendazole	100 mg bid x 3d
	OR Pyrantel pamoate	11 mg/kg once (max. 1 gram)
Alternative:	Piperazine citrate	75 mg/kg/d (max. 3.5 grams)/d x 2d
BABESIOSIS (Babesia sp)		
Drugs of choice:[12]	Clindamycin[7]	1.2 grams bid parenteral or 600 mg tid oral x 7d
	plus quinine	650 mg tid oral x 7d
BALANTIDIASIS (Balantidium coli)		
Drug of choice:	Tetracycline[7]	500 mg qid x 10d
Alternatives:	Iodoquinol[1,7]	650 mg tid x 20d
	Metronidazole[7]	750 mg tid x 5d
BLASTOCYSTIS hominis infection		
Drug of choice:	Iodoquinol[1]	650 mg tid x 20d
	OR Metronidazole	750 mg tid x 10d
CAPILLARIASIS (Capillaria philippinensis)		
Drug of choice:	Mebendazole[7]	200 mg bid x 20d
Alternative:	Thiabendazole[7]	25 mg/kg/d x 30d
Chagas' disease, see TRYPANOSOMIASIS		
Clonorchis sinensis, see FLUKE infection		
CRYPTOSPORIDIOSIS		
Cryptosporidium sp		
Drug of choice:[13]	Spiramycin	1 gram tid PO x 14d or more
CUTANEOUS LARVA MIGRANS (creeping eruption)		
Drug of choice:	Thiabendazole	25 mg/kg bid (max. 3 grams/d) x 2-5d and/or topically
Cysticercosis, see TAPEWORM infection		
DIENTAMOEBA fragilis infection		
Drug of choice:	Iodoquinol[1]	650 mg tid x 20d
	OR Tetracycline[7]	500 mg qid x 10d
	OR Paromomycin	25-30 mg/kg/d in 3 doses x 7d
Diphyllobothrium latum, see TAPEWORM infection		
DRACUNCULUS medinensis (guinea worm) infection		
Drug of choice:	Metronidazole[2,7]	250 mg tid x 10d
Alternative:	Thiabendazole[7]	25-37.5 mg/kg bid x 3d[11]
Echinococcus, see TAPEWORM infection		
Entamoeba histolytica, see AMEBIASIS		
ENTAMOEBA polecki infection		
Drugs of choice:	Metronidazole[3,7]	750 mg tid x 10d
	followed by	
	diloxanide furoate[2]	500 mg tid x 10d
ENTEROBIUS vermicularis (pinworm) infection		
Drug of choice:	Pyrantel pamoate	a single dose of 11 mg/kg (max. 1 gram); repeat after 2 weeks
	OR Mebendazole	A single dose of 100 mg; repeat after 2 weeks
Fasciola hepatica, see FLUKE infection		
FILARIASIS		
Wuchereria bancrofti, Brugia (W.) malayi, Mansonella ozzardi, Loa loa		
Drug of choice:[14]	Diethylcarbamazine[15]	Day 1: 50 mg, oral, p.c. Day 2: 50 mg tid Day 3: 100 mg tid Days 4 through 21: 2 mg/kg tid
Mansonella perstans		
Drug of choice:[16]	Mebendazole[7]	100 mg bid x 30d
Tropical eosinophilia		
Drug of choice:	Diethylcarbamazine	2 mg/kg tid x 7-10d

(continued)

104

Infection	Drug	Adult Dosage*
Filariasis *(continued)*		
Onchocerca volvulus		
Drug of choice:	Ivermectin[7,17]	150 µg/kg PO once, repeated every 6 to 12 months
Alternatives:	Diethylcarbamazine[15]	25 mg/d x 3d, then 50 mg/d x 5d, then 100 mg/d x 3d, then 150 mg/d x 12d
	followed by suramin[2,18]	100-200 mg (test dose) IV, then 1 gram IV at weekly intervals x 5 wks
FLUKE, hermaphroditic, infection		
Clonorchis sinensis (Chinese liver fluke)		
Drug of choice:	Praziquantel[7]	25 mg/kg tid x 2d
Fasciola hepatica (sheep liver fluke)		
Drugs of choice:[19]	Bithionol[2]	30-50 mg/kg on alternate days x 10-15 doses
Fasciolopsis buski (intestinal fluke)		
Drug of choice:	Praziquantel[7]	25 mg/kg tid x 1d
	OR Niclosamide[7]	a single dose of 4 tablets (2 g) chewed thoroughly
Alternative:	Tetrachloroethylene[20]	0.1 ml/kg (max. 5 ml)
Heterophyes heterophyes (intestinal fluke)		
Drug of choice:	Praziquantel[7]	25 mg/kg tid x 1d
Metagonimus yokogawai (intestinal fluke)		
Drug of choice:	Praziquantel[7]	25 mg/kg tid x 1d
Opisthorchis viverrini (liver fluke)		
Drug of choice:	Praziquantel[7]	25 mg/kg tid x 1d
Paragonimus westermani (lung fluke)		
Drug of choice:	Praziquantel[7]	25 mg/kg tid x 2d
Alternative:	Bithionol[2]	30-50 mg/kg on alternate days x 10-15 doses
GIARDIASIS (Giardia lamblia)		
Drug of choice:	Quinacrine HCl	100 mg tid p.c. x 5d
Alternatives:	Metronidazole[3,4,7]	250 mg tid x 5d
	Furazolidone	100 mg qid x 7-10d
GNATHOSTOMIASIS (Gnathostoma spinigerum)		
Treatment of choice:	Surgical removal	
	OR Mebendazole[7,21]	200 mg q3h x 6d
HOOKWORM infection (Ancylostoma duodenale, Necator americanus)		
Drug of choice:[22]	Mebendazole	100 mg bid x 3d
	OR Pyrantel pamoate[7]	11 mg/kg (max. 1 gram) x 3d
Hydatid cyst, see TAPEWORM infection		
Hymenolepis nana, see TAPEWORM infection		
ISOSPORIASIS (Isospora belli)		
Drug of choice:	Trimethoprim-sulfamethoxazole[7,23]	160 mg TMP, 800 mg SMX qid x 10d, then bid x 3 wks
LEISHMANIASIS		
L. braziliensis, L. mexicana (American cutaneous and mucocutaneous leishmaniasis)		
Drug of choice:[24]	Stibogluconate sodium[2]	20 mg/kg/d (max. 800 mg/d) IV or IM x 20d may be repeated or continued until there is a response
Alternative:	Amphotericin B[7]	0.25 to 1 mg/kg by slow infusion daily or every 2d for up to 8 wks

Infection	Drug	Adult Dosage*
Leishmaniasis (continued)		
L. donovani (kala azar, visceral leishmaniasis)		
Drug of choice:	Stibogluconate sodium[2,26]	20 mg/kg/d (max. 800 mg/d) IM or IV x 20d (may be repeated)
Alternative:	Pentamidine isethionate	2-4 mg/kg/d IM for up to 15 doses
L. tropica, L. major (oriental sore, cutaneous leishmaniasis)		
Drug of choice:	Stibogluconate sodium[2,26]	10 mg/kg/d (max. 600 mg/d) IM or IV x 6-10d (may be repeated)
Alternative:	Topical treatment[27]	
LICE infestation (Pediculus humanus, capitis, Phthirus pubis)[28]		
Drug of choice:	1% Permethrin[29]	Topically[30]
Alternatives:	Pyrethrins with piperonyl butoxide	Topically[30]
	Lindane	Topically[30]
Loa loa, see FILARIASIS		
MALARIA, see page 23		
Mites, see SCABIES		
Naegleria species, see AMEBIC MENINGOENCEPHALITIS, PRIMARY		
Necator americanus, see HOOKWORM infection		
Onchocerca volvulus, see FILARIASIS		
Opisthorchis viverrini, see FLUKE infection		
Paragonimus westermani, see FLUKE infection		
Pediculus capitis, humanus, Phthirus pubis, see LICE		
Pinworm, see ENTEROBIUS		
PNEUMOCYSTIS carinii pneumonia[31]		
Drug of choice:	Trimethoprim-sulfamethoxazole	TMP 20 mg/kg/d, SMX 100 mg/kg/d oral or IV in 4 doses x 14d
Alternative:	Pentamidine isethionate	4 mg/kg/d IM x 14d
Roundworm, see ASCARIASIS		
SCABIES (Sarcoptes scabiei)		
Drug of choice:[32]	Lindane	Topically once
Alternatives:	Sulfur in petrolatum	Topically
	10% Crotamiton	Topically
SCHISTOSOMIASIS		
S. haematobium		
Drug of choice:	Praziquantel	20 mg/kg tid x 1d
S. japonicum		
Drug of choice:	Praziquantel	20 mg/kg tid x 1d
S. mansoni		
Drug of choice:	Praziquantel	20 mg/kg tid x 1d
Alternative:	Oxamniquine	15 mg/kg once[33]
S. mekongi		
Drug of choice:	Praziquantel	20 mg/kg tid x 1d
Sleeping sickness, see TRYPANOSOMIASIS		

Infection	Drug	Adult Dosage*
STRONGYLOIDIASIS (Strongyloides stercoralis)		
Drug of choice:[34]	Thiabendazole	25 mg/kg bid (max. 3 grams/d) x 2d[35]
TAPEWORM infection — **Adult or intestinal stage**		
Diphyllobothrium latum (fish), Taenia saginata (beef), Taenia solium (pork),[36] Dipylidium caninum (dog)		
Drug of choice:[7]	Niclosamide	A single dose of 4 tablets (2 grams) chewed thoroughly
OR	Praziquantel[7]	10-20 mg/kg once
Hymenolepis nana (dwarf tapeworm)		
Drug of choice:[7]	Praziquantel[7]	25 mg/kg once
Alternative:	Niclosamide	A single daily dose of 4 tablets (2 grams) chewed thoroughly, then 2 tablets daily x 6d
— **Larval or tissue stage**		
Echinococcus granulosus (sheep, cattle, human, deer Hydatid cysts)		
Drug of choice:	See footnote 37	
Echinococcus multilocularis[38]		
Cysticercus cellulosae (cysticercosis)		
Drug of choice:[39]	Praziquantel[7]	50 mg/kg/d in 3 divided doses x 14d
Alternative:	Surgery	
Toxocariasis, see VISCERAL LARVA MIGRANS		
TOXOPLASMOSIS (Toxoplasma gondii)[40]		
Drugs of choice:	Pyrimethamine[41] **plus**	25 mg/d x 3-4 wks
	trisulfapyrimidines	2-6 grams/d x 3-4 wks
Alternative:	Spiramycin	2-4 grams/d x 3-4 wks
	Steroids for severe symptoms	
	plus thiabendazole[43]	
TRICHINOSIS (Trichinella spiralis)		
Drug of choice:		25 mg/kg bid x 5d (max. 3 grams/d)
TRICHOMONIASIS (Trichomonas vaginalis)		
Drug of choice:[44]	Metronidazole[3]	2 grams once or 250 mg tid orally x 7d
TRICHOSTRONGYLUS infection		
Drug of choice:	Thiabendazole[7]	25 mg/kg bid x 2d (max. 3 grams/d)
Alternative:	Pyrantel pamoate[7]	11 mg/kg once (max. 1 gram)
TRICHURIASIS (Trichuris trichura, whipworm)		
Drug of choice:	Mebendazole	100 mg bid x 3d

Infection	Drug	Adult Dosage*
TRYPANOSOMIASIS		
T. cruzi (South American trypanosomiasis, Chagas' disease)		
Drug of choice:	Nifurtimox[2]	8-10 mg/kg/d orally in 4 divided doses x 120d
Alternative:	Benznidazole[45]	5-7 mg/kg x 30-120d
T. gambiense; T. rhodesiense (African trypanosomiasis, sleeping sickness)		
hemolymphatic stage		
Drug of choice:[46]	Suramin[2]	100-200 mg (test dose) IV, then 1 gram IV on days 1,3,7,14, and 21
Alternative:	Pentamidine isethionate	4 mg/kg/d IM x 10d
late disease with CNS involvement		
Drug of choice:[46]	Melarsoprol[2,47]	2-3.6 mg/kg/d IV x 3 doses; after 1 wk 3.6 mg/kg/d IV x 3 doses; repeat again after 10-21 days
Alternatives:	Tryparsamide	One injection of 30 mg/kg IV every 5d to total of 12 injections; may be repeated after 1 mo.
	plus suramin[2]	One injection of 10 mg/kg IV every 5d to total of 12 injections; may be repeated after 1 mo.
VISCERAL LARVA MIGRANS[48]		
Drug of choice:[48]	Diethylcarbamazine[7]	2 mg/kg tid x 7-10d
	OR Thiabendazole[7]	25 mg/kg bid x 5d (max. 3 grams/d)
Alternative:	Mebendazole	200-400 mg/d x 5d[50]
Whipworm, see TRICHURIASIS		
Wuchereria bancrofti, see FILARIASIS		

* The letter indicates day.

1. Dosage and duration of administration should not be exceeded because of possibility of causing optic neuritis; maximum dosage is 2 grams/day.

2. In the USA, this drug is available from the CDC Drug Service, Centers for Disease Control, Atlanta, Georgia 30333; telephone: 404-639-3670 (evenings, weekends, and holidays: 404-639-2888).

3. Metronidazole is carcinogenic in rodents and mutagenic in bacteria; it should generally not be given to pregnant women, particularly in the first trimester.

4. Outside the USA, ornidazole and tinidazole are also used.

5. Dehydroemetine is probably as effective and probably less toxic than emetine. Because of its toxic effects on the heart, patients receiving emetine should have electrocardiographic monitoring and should remain sedentary during therapy.

6. One patient with a Naegleria infection was successfully treated with amphotericin B, miconazole, and rifampin (JS Seidel et al, N Engl J Med, 306:346, 1982).

7. Considered an investigational drug for this condition by the U.S. Food and Drug Administration.

8. Experimental infections with Acanthamoeba sp. have been reported to respond to sulfadiazine (CG Culbertson, Annu Rev Microbiol, 25:231, 1971). Amebic keratitis due to Acanthamoeba sp. has been reported to respond to topical miconazole, propamidine isethionate, and antibiotics (MB Moore et al, Am J Ophthalmol, 100:396, 1985).

9. Effectiveness documented only in animals.

10. Analgesics, corticosteroids, and careful removal of CSF at frequent intervals can relieve symptoms. Albendazole and ivermectin have been used successfully in animals.

11. This dose is likely to be toxic and may have to be decreased.

12. Concurrent use of pentamidine and trimethoprim-sulfamethoxazole has been reported to cure an infection with B. divergens (D Raoult et al, Ann Intern Med, 107:944, 1987).

13. Limited clinical results suggest a decrease in diarrhea with therapy. Infection is self-limiting in immunocompetent patients.

14. Several reports indicate that ivermectin may be effective for treatment of W. bancrofti (S Diallo et al, Lancet, 1:1030, 1987) and M. ozzardi (TB Nutman et al, J Infect Dis, 156:662, 1987).

15. Diethylcarbamazine should be administered with special caution in heavy infections with Loa loa because it can provoke ocular problems or an encephalopathy. Antihistamines or corticosteroids may be required to decrease allergic reactions due to disintegration of microfilariae in all filarial infections, especially those caused by Onchocerca and Loa loa. Surgical excision of subcutaneous Onchocerca nodules is recommended by some authorities before starting drug therapy.

16. Ivermectin may also be effective.

17. Ivermectin in a dose of 200 μg/kg has been reported to be as effective as diethylcarbamazine in decreasing the number of microfilaria and causes fewer adverse ophthalmologic reactions (BM Greene et al, N Engl J Med, 313:133, 1985; AT White et al, J Infect Dis, 156:463, 1987). Semiannual to annual prophylaxis appears to be effective in keeping microfilarial counts at low levels.

18. Some Medical Letter consultants use suramin only if ocular microfilariae persist after diethylcarbamazine therapy and nodulectomy.

19. Unlike infections with other flukes, fasciola hepatica infections may not respond to praziquantel. Limited data indicate that albendazole may be effective in this condition.

20. Given on empty stomach. Although approved for human use, it is available currently only as a veterinary product. No alcoholic beverage should be consumed before or for 12 hours after therapy. Keep patient at bedrest for 4 hours after treatment.

21. In felines, ancylol (2, 6, diodo-4-nitrophenol) by subcutaneous injection has been effective against migrating larvae.

22. Albendazole is also effective (RNG Pugh, Ann Trop Med Parasitol, 80:665, 1986).

23. In sulfonamide-sensitive patients, such as AIDS, pyrimethamine 50-75 mg daily has been effective. In immunocompromised patients, it may be necessary to continue therapy indefinitely.

24. Limited data indicate that ketoconazole, 400 to 600 mg daily for 28 days, may be effective for treatment of L. panamensis and L. mexicana (cutaneous).

25. For the African form of visceral leishmaniasis, therapy may have to be extended to at least 30 days and may have to be repeated.

26. Ketoconazole, 400 mg daily four to eight weeks, has also been reported to be effective (J Viallet et al, Am J Trop Med Hyg, 35:491, 1986).

27. Application of heat 39° to 42°C directly to the lesion for 20 to 32 hours over a period of 10 to 12 days has been reported to be effective in L. tropica minor (FA Neva et al, Am J Trop Med Hyg, 33:800, 1984).

28. For infestation of eyelashes with crab lice, use petrolatum.
29. FDA-approved for head lice only
30. Some consultants recommend a second application one week later to kill hatching progeny.
31. AIDS patients may need longer duration of therapy. For AIDS patients who develop hypersensitivity or resistance to both TMP/SMX and pentamidine, trimetrexate with leucovorin rescue or a combination of dapsone and trimethoprim may be effective. Aerosolized pentamidine has been tried for both treatment and prophylaxis (Medical Letter, 29:103, 1987).
32. 5% permethrin, not yet marketed in the USA, could prove to be the drug of choice when it becomes available.
33. In East Africa, the dose should be increased to 30 mg/kg/d, and in Egypt and South Africa, 30 mg/kg/d x 2d. Neuropsychiatric disturbances and seizures have been reported in some patients (H Stokvis et al, Am J Trop Med Hyg, 35:330, 1986).
34. Albendazole or ivermectin have also been effective.
35. In disseminated strongyloidiasis, thiabendazole therapy should be continued for at least five days. In immunocompromised patients it may be necessary to continue therapy or use other agents (see footnote 34).
36. Niclosamide is effective for the treatment of T. solium but, since it causes disintegration of segments and release of viable eggs, its use creates a theoretical risk of causing cysticercosis. It should therefore be followed in three or four hours by a purge. Quinacrine is preferred by some clinicians because it expels T. solium intact.
37. Surgical resection of cysts is the treatment of choice. When surgery is contraindicated, or cysts rupture spontaneously during surgery, mebendazole (experimental for this purpose in the USA) can be tried (JF Wilson and RL Rausch, Ann Trop Med Parasitol, 76:165, 1982; ADM Bryceson et al, Trans R Soc Trop Med Hyg, 76:510, 1982). Albendazole has also been reported to be effective (DL Morris et al, JAMA, 253:2053, 1985). Flubendazole has also been used with some success (E Tellez-Giron et al, Am J Trop Med Hyg, 33:627, 1984). Praziquantel and albendazole will kill protoscolices and may be useful in case of spill during surgery.
38. Surgical excision is the only reliable means of treatment although recent reports have been encouraging about use of albendazole or mebendazole (JF Wilson et al, Am J Trop Med Hyg, 37:162, 1987; A Davis et al, Bull WHO, 64:383, 1986). .
39. Corticosteroids should be given for two to three days before and during praziquantel therapy. Praziquantel should not be used for ocular or spinal cord cysticercosis. Metrifonate 7.5 mg/kg x 5d, repeated six times at two-week intervals, has been reported to be effective for ocular as well as cerebral and subcutaneous disease. Albendazole, 15 mg/kg x 30d, which can be repeated, has been used successfully (F Escobedo et al, Arch Intern Med, 147:738, 1987).
40. In ocular toxoplasmosis, corticosteroids should also be used for anti-inflammatory effect on the eyes.
41. Pyrimethamine is teratogenic in animals. To prevent hematological toxicity from pyrimethamine, it is advisable to give leucovorin (folinic acid), about 10 mg/day, either by injection or orally. Pyrimethamine alone 50-75 mg daily has been used to treat CNS toxoplasmosis after sulfonamide sensitivity develops. In AIDS patients treatment should continue indefinitely.
42. Every two to three days for infants. Most authorities would treat congenitally infected newborns for about one year.
43. The efficacy of thiabendazole for trichinosis is not clearly established; it appears to be effective during the intestinal phase but its effect on larvae that have migrated is questionable. In the tissue phase, mebendazole 200-400 mg tid x 3 days, then 400-500 mg tid x 10 days, may be effective. Albendazole may also be effective for this indication.
44. Sexual partners should be treated simultaneously. Outside the USA, ornidazole and tinidazole have been used for this condition. Metronidazole-resistant strains have been reported; higher doses of metronidazole for longer periods of time are sometimes effective against these strains.
45. Limited data
46. In drug-resistant cases of T. gambiense infections, eflornithine (difluoromethylornithine, Merrell Dow) has been used successfully; field trials are now underway (H Taelman et al, Am J Med, 82:607, 1987; F Doua et al, Am J Trop Med Hyg, 37:525, 1987; J Pepin et al, Lancet, 2:1431, 1987). It is highly effective in both CNS and non-CNS infections with T. gambiense.
47. In frail patients, begin with as little as 18 mg and increase the dose progressively. Pretreatment with suramin has been advocated for debilitated patients.
48. For severe symptoms or eye involvement, corticosteroids can be used in addition.
49. Ivermectin and albendazole have been effective in some animal studies.
50. One report of a cure using 1 gram tid for 21 days has been published (A Bekhti, Ann Intern Med, 100:463, 1984).

Malaria Prophylaxis and Treatment (MMWR 37:277,1988)

<u>Malaria prevention information system</u>: CDC information available 24 hr/day at (404) 639-1610 (MMWR 37:336,1988).

<u>Risk areas</u>: Large areas of Central and South America, Sub-Saharan Africa, Indian subcontinent, Southeast Asia (Thailand, Indonesia, Malaysia, China, Philippines, Burma, Kampuchea, Vietnam, Laos), Middle East and Oceania. Relative risk for <u>P. falciparum</u> malaria is greatest for Sub-Saharan Africa.

<u>Drug resistant P. falciparum</u>: Resistance to chloroquine in all countries <u>except</u>: Dominican Republic, Haiti, Central America, Middle East and parts of West Africa (Chad, Equatorial Guinea, Guinea, Guinea-Bissau, Liberia, Senegal, Sierra Leone) Resistance to chloroquine and Fansidar is widespread in Thailand, Berma, Kampuchea.

General advice

1) Transmission is most common from dusk to dawn.

2) Protective measures include screened areas, clothing, mosquito nets; insect repellents for skin should contain N,N diethylmetatoluamide (DEET), preferably in large concentrations; insect sprays for living areas should contain pyrethrum.

Chemoprophylaxis

1. Areas with no or only low levels of chloroquine-resistant <u>P. falciparum</u> (CRPF): Chloroquine (500 mg po once weekly) beginning 1-2 weeks prior to travel through 4 weeks post departure from malarious area. Intolerance may be reduced by taking with meals, dividing dose (250 twice weekly) or use of hydroxychloroquine.

2. Areas where CRPF is endemic: Chloroquine alone; additionally, a supply of Fansidar (3 tabs) is provided to be taken for a febrile illness if professional medical care is not available. Doxycycline (100 mg po daily) is an alternative in CRPF endemic areas, especially for those with sulfonamide reactions (Fansidar contraindicated) and for travel to areas with Fansidar resistance (forested areas of Thailand, Burma, Kampuchea). Doxycycline should be started 1-2 days prior to travel and should be continued through 4 weeks post travel in malarious areas. Fansidar (1 tab weekly) plus chloroquine may be used prophylactically in areas of high risk, but traveler should be warned of adverse reactions.

3. Primaquine: To prevent relapse of <u>P. vivax</u> and <u>P. ovale</u>. Most malarious areas have these species, but primaquine prophylaxis is usually restricted to those with prolonged exposure, eg., missionaries and Peace Corps volunteers. Primaquine is given (15 mg base po once daily x 2 weeks) for last 2 weeks of chloroquine prophylaxis after leaving malarious area.

4. Pregnancy; **a)** Chloroquine-considered safe; **b)** Fansidar - safety not clearly established (pyrimethamine is teratogenic in animals, but there is no evidence it is a human teratogen; sulfadoxine could exacerbate neonatal jaundice); **c)** Doxycycline is contraindicated.

111

Drug	Prophylaxis		Presumptive Treatment for Travelers to Areas of Chloroquine Resistance	
	Adult Dose	Pediatric Dose		
Chloroquine phosphate (Aralen®*)	300 mg base (500 mg salt) orally, once/week	5 mg/kg base (8.3 mg/kg salt) orally, once/week, up to maximum adult dose of 300 mg base	Chloroquine is not recommended for the presumptive treatment of malaria acquired in areas of known chloroquine resistance.	
Hydroxy-chloroquine sulfate (Plaquenil®*)	310 mg base (400 mg salt) orally, once/week	5 mg/kg base (6.5 mg/kg salt) orally, once/week, up to maximum adult dose of 310 mg base	Hydroxychloroquine is not recommended for the presumptive treatment of malaria acquired in areas of known chloroquine resistance.	
Doxycycline	100 mg orally, once/day	>8 years of age: 2 mg/kg of body weight orally, once/day up to adult dose of 100 mg/day	Tetracyclines are not recommended for the presumptive treatment of malaria.	
Proguanil (Paludrine®*)	200 mg orally, once/day, in combination with weekly chloroquine	<2 yrs: 50 mg/day 2–6 yrs: 100 mg/day 7–10 yrs: 150 mg/day >10 yrs: 200 mg/day	Proguanil is not recommended for the presumptive treatment of malaria.	
Pyrimethamine-sulfadoxine (Fansidar®*)	1 tablet (25 mg pyrimethamine and 500 mg sulfadoxine) orally, once/week	2–11 mos: ⅛ tab/wk 1–3 yrs: ¼ tab/wk 4–8 yrs: ½ tab/wk 9–14 yrs: ¾ tab/wk >14 yrs: 1 tab/wk	**Adult Dose** 3 tablets (75 mg pyrimethamine and 1,500 mg sulfa-doxine), orally, as a single dose	**Pediatric Dose** 2–11 mos: ¼ tab 1–3 yrs: ½ tab 4–8 yrs: 1 tab 9–14 yrs: 2 tabs >14 yrs: 3 tabs as a single dose
Primaquine	15 mg base (26.3 mg salt) orally, once/day for 14 days, or 45 mg base (79 mg salt) orally, once/week for 8 weeks	0.3 mg/kg base (0.5 mg/kg salt) orally, once/day for 14 days, or 0.9 mg/kg base (1.5 mg/kg salt) orally, once/week for 8 weeks	Primaquine is only recommended for use after leaving an endemic area to prevent relapses of *Plasmodium vivax* and *P. ovale*.	

*Use of trade names is for identification only and does not imply endorsement by the U.S. Department of Health and Human Services or the Public Health Service.

AIDS

A. Case Definition for Acquired Immunodeficiency Syndrome (Center for Disease Control, MMWR 36:3S,1987)

For national reporting, a case of AIDS is defined as an illness characterized by one or more of the following "indicator" diseases, depending on the status of laboratory evidence of HIV infection, as shown below.

I. Without Laboratory Evidence Regarding HIV infection

If laboratory tests for HIV were not performed or gave inconclusive results (See Appendix I) and the patient had no other cause of immunodeficiency listed in Section I.A below, then any disease listed in Section I.B indicates AIDS if it was diagnosed by a definitive method (See Appendix II).

A. Causes of immunodeficiency that disqualify diseases as indicators of AIDS in the absence of laboratory evidence for HIV infection

1. high-dose or long-term systemic corticosteroid therapy or other immunosuppressive/cytotoxic therapy ≤ 3 months before the onset of the indicator disease

2. any of the following diseases diagnosed ≤ 3 months after diagnosis of the indicator disease: Hodgkin's disease, non-Hodgkin's lymphoma (other than primary brain lymphoma), lymphocytic leukemia, multiple myeloma, any other cancer of lymphoreticular or histiocytic tissue, or angioimmunoblastic lymphadenopathy

3. a genetic (congenital) immunodeficiency syndrome or an acquired immunodeficiency syndrome atypical of HIV infection, such as one involving hypogammaglobulinemia

B. Indicator diseases diagnosed definitively (See Appendix II)

1. candidiasis of the esophagus, trachea, bronchi, or lungs
2. cryptococcosis, extrapulmonary
3. cryptosporidiosis with diarrhea persisting > 1 month
4. cytomegalovirus disease of an organ other than liver, spleen, or lymph nodes in a patient > 1 month of age
5. herpes simplex virus infection causing a mucocutaneous ulcer that persists longer than 1 month; or bronchitis pneumonitis, or esophagitis for any duration affecting a patient > 1 month of age
6. Kaposi's sarcoma affecting a patient < 60 years of age
7. lymphoma of the brain (primary) affecting a patient < 60 years of age
8. lymphoid interstitial pneumonia and/or pulmonary lymphoid hyperplasia (LIP/PLH complex) affecting a child < 13 years of age
9. Mycobacterium avium complex or M kansasii disease, disseminated (at a site other than or in addition to lungs, skin, or cervical or hilar lymph nodes)
10. Pneumocystis carinii pneumonia
11. progressive multifocal leukoencephalopathy
12. toxoplasmosis of the brain affecting a patient > 1 month of age

II. With Laboratory Evidence for HIV Infection

Regardless of the presence of other causes of immunodeficiency (I.A), in the presence of laboratory evidence for HIV infection (See Appendix I), any disease listed above (I.B) or below (II.A or II.B) indicates a diagnosis of AIDS.

A. Indicator diseases diagnosed definitively (See Appendix II)

1. bacterial infections, multiple or recurrent (any combination of at least two within a 2-year period), of the following types affecting a child < 13 years of age:

   septicemia, pneumonia, meningitis, bone or joint infection, or abscess of an internal organ or body cavity (excluding otitis media or superficial skin or mucosal abscesses), caused by Haemophilus, Streptococcus (including pneumococcus), or other pyogenic bacteria

2. coccidioidomycosis, disseminated (at a site other than or in addition to lungs or cervical or hilar lymph nodes)

3. HIV encephalopathy (also called "HIV dementia," "AIDS dementia," or "subacute encephalitis due to HIV") (See Appendix II for description)

4. histoplasmosis, disseminated (at a site other than or in addition to lungs or cervical or hilar lymph nodes)

5. isosporiasis with diarrhea persisting > 1 month

6. Kaposi's sarcoma at any age

7. lymphoma of the brain (primary) at any age

8. other non-Hodgkin's lymphoma of B-cell or unknown immunologic phenotype and the following histologic types):

   a. small noncleaved lymphoma (either Burkitt or non-Burkitt type)

   b. immunoblastic sarcoma (equivalent to any of the following, although not necessarily all in combination: immunoblastic lymphoma, large-cell lymphoma, diffuse histiocytic lymphoma, diffuse undifferentiated lymphoma, or high-grade lymphoma)

   Note: Lymphomas are not included here if they are of T-cell immunologic phenotype or their histologic type is not described or is described as "lymphocytic", "lymphoblastic", "small cleaved", or "plasmacytoid lymphocytic"

9. any mycobacterial disease caused by mycobacteria other than M. tuberculosis, disseminated (at a site other than or in addition to lungs, skin, or cervical or hilar lymph nodes)

10. disease caused by M. tuberculosis, extrapulmonary (involving at least one site outside the lungs, regardless of whether there is concurrent pulmonary involvement)

11. Salmonella (nontyphoid) septicemia, recurrent

12. HIV wasting syndrome (emaciation, "slim disease") (See Appendix II for description)

B. Indicator diseases diagnosed presumptively (by a method other than those in Appendix II)

Note: Given the seriousness of diseases indicative of AIDS, it is generally important to diagnose them definitively, especially when therapy that would be used may have serious side effects or when definitive diagnosis is needed for eligibility for antiretroviral therapy. Nonetheless, in some situations, a patient's condition will not permit the performance of definitive tests. In other situations, accepted clinical practice may be to diagnose presumptively based on the presence of characteristic clinical and laboratory abnormalities. Guidelines for presumptive diagnoses are suggested in Appendix III.

1. candidiasis of the esophagus
2. cytomegalovirus retinitis with loss of vision
3. Kaposi's sarcoma
4. lymphoid interstitial pneumonia and/or pulmonary lymphoid hyperplasia (LIP/PLH complex) affecting a child < 13 years of age
5. mycobacterial disease (acid-fast bacilli with species not identified by culture), disseminated (involving at least one site other than or in addition to lungs, skin, or cervical or hilar lymph nodes)
6. <u>Pneumocystis carinii</u> pneumonia
7. toxoplasmosis of the brain affecting a patient > 1 month of age

III. **With Laboratory Evidence Against HIV Infection**

   With laboratory test results negative for HIV infection (See Appendix I), a diagnosis of AIDS for surveillance purposes is ruled out unless:

   A. all the other causes of immunodeficiency listed above in Section I.A are excluded; **AND**

   B. the patient has had either:
      1. <u>Pneumocystis carinii</u> pneumonia diagnosed by a definitive method (See Appendix II); **OR**
      2. **a.** any of the other diseases indicative of AIDS listed above in Section I.B diagnosed by a definitive method (See Appendix II); **AND**
         b. a T-helper/inducer (CD4) lymphocyte count < 400/mm^3.

APPENDIX I

Laboratory Evidence For or Against HIV Infection

1. **For Infection:**
   When a patient has disease consistent with AIDS:

   a. a serum specimen from a patient ≥ 15 months of age, or from a child < 15 of age whose mother is not thought to have had HIV infection during the child's perinatal period, that is repeatedly reactive for HIV antibody by a screening test (e.g., enzyme-linked immunosorbent assay [ELISA]), as long as subsequent HIV-antibody tests (e.g., Western blot, immunofluorescence assay), if done, are positive; **OR**

   b. a serum specimen from a child < 15 months of age, whose mother is thought to have had HIV infection during the child's perinatal period, that is repeatedly reactive for HIV antibody by a screening test (e.g., ELISA), plus increased serum immunoglobulin levels and at least one of the following abnormal immunologic test results: reduced absolute lymphocyte count, depressed CD4 (T-helper) lymphocyte count, or decreased CD4/CD8 (helper/suppressor) ratio, as long as subsequent antibody tests (e.g., Western blot, immunofluorescence assay), if done, are positive; **OR**

   c. a positive test for HIV serum antigen; **OR**

   d. a positive HIV culture confirmed by both reverse transcriptase detection and a specific HIV-antigen test or in situ hybridization using a nucleic acid probe; **OR**

   e. a positive result on any other highly specific test for HIV (e.g., nucleic acid probe of peripheral blood lymphocytes).

2. **Against Infection:**

   A nonreactive screening test for serum antibody to HIV (e.g., ELISA) without a reactive or positive result on any other test for HIV infection (e.g., antibody, antigen, culture), if done.

3. **Inconclusive (Neither For nor Against Infection):**

   a. a repeatedly reactive screening test for serum antibody to HIV (e.g., ELISA) followed by a negative or inconclusive supplemental test (e.g., Western blot, immunofluorescence assay) without a positive HIV culture or serum antigen test, if done; **OR**

   b. a serum specimen from a child < 15 months of age, whose mother is thought to have had HIV infection during the child's perinatal period, that is repeatedly reactive for HIV antibody by a screening test, even if positive by a supplemental test, without additional evidence for immunodeficiency as described above (in I.b) and without a positive HIV culture or serum antigen test, if done.

APPENDIX II

Definitive Diagnostic Methods for Disease Indicative of AIDS

Diseases	Definitive Diagnostic Methods
cryptosporidiosis cytomegalovirus isosporiasis Kaposi's sarcoma lymphoma lymphoid pneumonia or hyperplasia Pneumocystis carinii pneumonia progressive multifocal leukoencephalopathy toxoplasmosis	microscopy (histology or cytology).
candidiasis	gross inspection by endoscopy or autopsy or by microscopy (histology or cytology) on a specimen obtained directly from the tissues affected (including scrapings from the mucosal surface), not from a culture.
coccidioidomycosis	microscopy (histology or cytology), culture, or detection of antigen in a specimen obtained directly from the tissues affected or a fluid from those tissues.
tuberculosis other mycobacteriosis salmonellosis other bacterial infection	culture.
HIV encephalopathy* (dementia)	clinical findings of disabling cognitive and/or motor dysfunction interfering with occupation or activities of daily living, or loss of behavioral developmental milestones affecting a child, progressing over weeks to months, in the absence of a concurrent illness or condition other than HIV infection that could explain the findings. Methods to rule out such concurrent illnesses and conditions must include cerebrospinal fluid examination and either brain imaging (computed tomography or magnetic resonance) or autopsy.
HIV wasting syndrome*	findings of profound involuntary weight loss <10% of baseline body weight plus either chronic diarrhea (at least two loose stools per day for ≥ 30 days) or chronic weakness and documented fever (for ≥ 30 days, intermittent or constant) in the absence of a concurrent illness or condition other than HIV that could explain the findings (e.g., cancer, tuberculosis, cryptosporidiosis, or other specific enteritis).

*For HIV encephalopathy and HIV wasting syndrome, the methods of diagnosis described here are
not truly definitive, but are sufficiently rigorous for surveillance purposes.

APPENDIX III

Suggested Guidelines for Presumptive Diagnosis of Diseases Indicative of AIDS

Diseases	Presumptive Diagnostic Criteria
candidiasis of esophagus	a. recent onset of retrosternal pain on swallowing; AND b. oral candidiasis diagnosed by the gross appearance of white patches or plaques on an erythematous base or by the microscopic appearance of fungal mycelial filaments in an uncultured specimen scraped from the oral mucosa.
cytomegalovirus retinitis	a characteristic appearance on serial ophthalmoscopic examinations (e.g., discrete patches of retinal whitening with distinct borders, spreading in a centrifugal manner, following blood vessels, progressing over several months, frequently associated with retinal vasculitis, hemorrhage, and necrosis). Resolution of active disease leaves retinal scarring and atrophy with retinal pigment epithelial mottling.
mycobacteriosis	microscopy of a specimen from stool or normally sterile body fluids or tissue from a site other than lungs, skin, or cervical or hilar lymph nodes, showing acid-fast bacilli of a species not identified by culture.
Kaposi's sarcoma	a characteristic gross appearance of an erythematous or violaceous plaque-like lesion on skin or mucous membrane. (Note: Presumptive diagnosis of Kaposi's sarcoma should not be made by clinicians who have seen few cases of it.)
lymphoid interstitial pneumonia	bilateral reticulonodular interstitial pulmonary infiltrates present on chest x ray for ≥ 2 months with no pathogen identified and no response to antibiotic treatment.
Pneumocystis carinii pneumonia	a. a history of dyspnea on exertion or nonproductive cough of recent onset (within the past 3 months); AND b. chest x-ray evidence of diffuse bilateral interstitial infiltrates or gallium scan evidence of diffuse bilateral pulmonary disease; AND c. arterial blood gas analysis showing an arterial pO_2 of <70 mm Hg or a low respiratory diffusing capacity (<80% of predicted values) or an increase in the alveolar-arterial oxygen tension gradient; AND d. no evidence of a bacterial pneumonia.
toxoplasmosis of the brain	a. recent onset of a focal neurologic abnormality consistent with intracranial disease or a reduced level of consciousness; AND b. brain imaging evidence of a lesion having a mass effect (on computed tomography or nuclear magnetic resonance) or the radiographic appearance of which is enhanced by injection of contrast medium; AND c. serum antibody to toxoplasmosis or successful response to therapy for toxoplasmosis.

B. Recommendations for HIV Serologic Testing (MMWR 36:509,1987)

"Guidelines are based on public health considerations for HIV testing, including the principles of counseling before and after testing, confidentiality or personal information, and understanding that a person may decline to be tested without being denied health care or other services except where testing is required by law". Specific recommendations:

1. Persons who have sexually transmitted diseases.

2. IV drug abusers.

3. Persons who consider themselves at risk.

4. Women at risk who are of child bearing age or pregnant. Risk categories are: IV drug abuse; prostitution; male sexual partners who are bisexual, IV drug abusers or HIV infected; living in communities or born in countries with high prevalence in women, and blood transfusion between 1978-1985.

5. Prostitutes (male and female).

6. Medical evaluation (diagnostic test) for patients with selected clinical findings including generalized lymphadenopathy; unexplained dementia; chronic, unexplained fever or diarrhea; unexplained weight loss; or diseases such as tuberculosis, sexually transmitted diseases, generalized herpes, chronic candidiasis, other opportunistic infections suggesting unexplained defective cell-mediated immunity*, unexplained cytopenias* (anemia, leukopenia, lymphopenia, thrombocytopenia) and unexplained neurologic syndromes* (Guillain-Barre syndrome, aseptic meningitis, peripheral neuropathies).

7. Pregnant women, especially in high incidence areas*

8. Patients with tuberculosis, especially if severe, extrapulmonary or unusual in presentation, or if patient is in risk category.

9. Recipient and source of blood or body fluid exposures*. Body fluids considered at risk include: semen, vaginal secretions, cerebrospinal fluids, synovial fluid, pleural fluid, peritoneal fluid, pericardial fluid, amniotic fluid and any bloody body fluid. Body fluids not considered at risk are feces, nasal secretions, sputum, saliva, sweat, tears, urine and vomitus unless they contain visible blood (MMWR 37:377,1988).

10. "Consideration categories" depending on seroprevalence, cost-effectiveness, implementation process, etc: persons considering marriage, hospital admissions (age group with high incidence and persons in correctional systems.

* Added by author

119

C. Management of Opportunistic Infections in Patients with HIV Infection

	Preferred	Alternative	Comment
PROTOZOA			
Pneumocystis carinii			
Acute infection	Trimethoprim (15-20 mg/kg/day) + sulfamethoxazole (75-100 mg/kg/day) po or IV x 14-21 days in 3-4 daily doses	Pentamidine (4 mg/kg/day) IV (or IM)	Alternatives for patients with mild illness: 1) Aerosolized pentamidine (600 mg/day) x 14-21 days 2) Dapsone (100 mg q 24 h) + Trimethoprim (5 mg/kg q 6 h) po x 14-21 days Failure to respond to standard regimen: 1) Switch from trimethoprim-sulfa to pentamidine (or vice versa) 2) Add pentamidine 3) Change to trimetrexate (experimental) (45 mg/m^2 q 24 h) IV 4) Add corticosteroids (Solu-medrol, 50-500 mg IV q 6 h x 1-10 days)
Prophylaxis	1. Aerosolized pentamidine (300 mg) q month 2. Trimethoprim (5 mg/kg) + sulfamethoxazole (20 mg/kg) po (1 DS) q 12 h q d or 2-3 x/wk. 3. Pyrimethamine (25 mg) + sulfadoxine (500 mg) po q wk (1 Fansidar/wk)		Relative merits of these regimens are unknown Prophylaxis is indicated for any AIDS patient with a history of pneumocystis pneumonia; indications in other settings are not clearly defined

	Preferred	Alternative	Comment
	4. Dapsone (100 mg) po q d + trimethoprim (320 mg) po bid 5. Pentamidine (4 mg/kg) IV q month		
Toxoplasma encephalitis Acute infection	Pyrimethamine (25-75 mg/day) po + folinic acid (5-15 mg/day) po + sulfadiazine or trisulfa-pyrimidines (4-8 gm/day) po for at least 6 wks	Pyrimethamine + folinic acid (prior doses) + clindamycin (900-1200 mg) IV q 6-8 h for at least 6 weeks	All patients who respond to primary therapy should receive lifelong suppressive therapy
Suppressive therapy	Pyrimethamine (25 mg) po q d plus sulfadiazine or trisulfapyrimidines (2-4 gm/day) po q d or 3-5 x/week	Pyrimethamine (25 mg) po qd plus clindamycin (300-450 mg) po q 6-8 h	
Cryptosporidia	Spiramycin (experimental) (1 gm) po tid		Efficacy of spiramycin is not established
Isospora Acute infection	Trimethoprim (5 mg/kg) + sulfamethoxazole po bid (2 DS po bid) x 1 month		Duration of high dose therapy is not well defined
Suppressive treatment	Trimethoprim (2.5 mg/kg) + sulfamethoxazole (1-2 x/day) po	Pyrimethamine (25 mg) + sulfadoxine (500 mg) po q wk (1 Fansidar/wk)	Duration is not well defined

	Preferred	Alternative	Comment
FUNGI			
<u>Candida</u>			
Thrush			
Initial infection	Nystatin (500,000 units qid) orally. Clotrimazole oral troches (10 mg) qid	Ketoconazole (200 mg) po bid; amphotericin B (0.3-0.5 mg/kg) IV q day	Treat until symptoms resolve and then begin maintenance therapy
Maintenance treatment	Nystatin (above doses), clotrimazole (above doses) or ketoconazole 200 mg q d or bid		
Esophagitis			
Initial infection	Ketoconazole (200 mg) po bid or tid	Amphotericin B (0.3-0.5 mg/kg) IV q day $\pm$ flucytosine (100 mg/kg/day) x 5-7 days	
Maintenance	Ketoconazole (200 mg) po 1-2 x/day		
<u>Cryptococcal meningitis</u>			
Initial treatment	Amphotericin B (0.4-0.6 mg/kg/day) IV with or without 5-flucytosine (75-100 mg/kg/day) po in 6 doses x 6-10 wks	Fluconazole (experimental) (200-400 mg/day) po	Duration of initial therapy is influenced by CSF cultures and Ag assay
Maintenance therapy	Amphotericin B (1 mg/kg/wk)	Fluconazole (experimental) (200 mg) po qd or bid	Maintenance therapy is life long

	Preferred	Alternative	Comment
Histoplasmosis Disseminated Initial treatment	Amphotericin B 2-2.5 gm (total dose)		
Maintenance	Amphotericin B (1 mg/kg/wk) or Ketoconazole (200 mg) po bid		
Coccidioidomycosis	Same as histoplasmosis		
MYCOBACTERIA M. tuberculosis	INH (300 mg) po + rifampin (600 mg) po + pyrazinamide (20-30 mg/kg) po/day x 2 months; then INH + rifampin (above doses) for at least 9 months total therapy and 6 months post culture conversion	INH + rifampin + streptomycin (0.75-1.0 mg/kg/day IM) x 2 mo., then INH + rifampin	Ethambutol (25 mg/kg/day) should be included in the initial (2 months) of therapy if CNS, disseminated disease or INH resistance is suspected. INH prophylaxis for ≥ 1 yr is indicated for all HIV infected patients with + PPD and no evidence of active disease
M. avium-intracellulare	Clofazimine (50-60 mg/day), ethambutol (25 mg/kg/day), rifampin (600 mg/day) ± amikacin (7.5 mg/kg IM or IV q 12 h for 4-8 wks)	Other combinations including INH, ethionamide, ansamycin (in place of rifampin), cycloserine, pyrazinamide, ciprofloxacine, imipenem	Efficacy of any treatment regimen is not established

	Preferred	Alternative	Comment
VIRUSES			
<u>Herpes simplex</u>			
Mucocutaneous			
Initial treatment			
Mild	Acyclovir (200-400 mg) po 5 x/day at least 10 days (until lesions crusted)		Failure to respond: double oral dose or give IV
Severe	Acyclovir (15 mg/kg/day) IV		If fails to respond give 30 mg/kg/day and test sensitivity of isolates to acyclovir
Maintenance	Acyclovir (200 mg) po tid		
Visceral	Acyclovir (30 mg/kg/day) IV at least 10 days	Vidarabine (15 mg/kg) IV x 10 days	
<u>Herpes zoster</u>			
Dermatomal	Acyclovir (30 mg/kg/day) IV at least 7 days (until lesions crust)	Acyclovir (800 mg) po 5 x/day	Corticosteroids should be avoided Postherpetic neuralgia is unusual No maintenance therapy recommended
Disseminated or visceral	Acyclovir (30 mg/kg/day) IV at least 7 days		
<u>Cytomegalovirus</u>			
Retinitis			
Initial treatment	Ganciclovir (experimental) (5 mg/kg) IV bid x 14 days	Foscarnet (experimental) (60 mg/kg) IV q8h x 14 d	Efficacy established for ganciclovir
Maintenance	Ganciclovir (experimental) (5 mg/kg) IV q d	Foscarnet (experimental) (90 mg/kg) IV qd	Maintenance therapy may be required life long

124

	Preferred	Alternative	Comment
Enteritis, colitis, esophagitis, pneumonitis	Ganciclovir (experimental) (5 mg/kg) IV bid x 14 days		Efficacy not clearly established Indications for maintenance therapy not established
BACTERIA			
<u>S. pneumoniae</u>	Penicillin	Erythromycin Cephalosporins	Traditional therapy usually adequate
<u>H. influenzae</u>	Cefuroxime/cefamandole Ampicillin/amoxicillin	Trimethoprim- sulfamethoxazole Cephalosporins - 3rd generation	Traditional therapy usually adequate
Salmonella Acute	Ampicillin (8-12 gm/day) IV x 1-4 wks; then amoxicillin (500 mg) po tid to complete 2-4 wk course Ciprofloxacin (500-750) mg po bid x 2-4 wks)	Trimethoprim (5-10 mg/ kg/day) + sulfamethoxa- zole IV or po x 4 wks. Cephalosporins - 3rd generation	Relapse common
Maintenance	Amoxicillin (250 mg) po bid	Ciprofloxacin (500 mg) po q d or bid. Trimethoprim + sulfamethoxazole (2.5 mg/kg trimethoprim or 1 DS) po bid.	Indications for maintenance therapy, specific regimens and duration not well defined

PATHOGENS ASSOCIATED WITH IMMUNODEFICIENCY STATUS

Condition	Usual conditions	Pathogens
Neutropenia (< 500/ml)	Cancer chemotherapy; Adverse drug reaction; Leukemia	Bacteria: Aerobic GNB (coliforms and pseudomonads) Fungi: Aspergillus, Phycomycetes
Cell-mediated immunity	Organ transplantation; HIV infection; Lymphoma (especially Hodgkin's disease); Cortico-steroid therapy	Bacteria: Listeria, Salmonella, Nocardia, Mycobacteria (M. tuberculosis & M. avium), Legionella Viruses: CMV, H. simplex, Varicella-zoster Parasites: Pneumocystis carinii; Toxoplasma; Strongyloides stercoralis; Cryptosporidia Fungi: Candida, Phycomycetes (Mucor), Cryptococcus
Hypogammaglobulinemia or dysgamma-globulinemia	Multiple myeloma; Congenital or acquired deficiency; Chronic lymphocytic leukemia	Bacteria: S. pneumoniae, H. influenzae (type B) Parasites: Giardia Viruses: Enteroviruses
Complement deficiencies C2, 3	Congenital	Bacteria S. pneumoniae, H. influenzae
C5		S. pneumoniae, S. aureus Enterobacteriaceae
C6-8		Neisseria meningitidis
Alternative pathway		S. pneumoniae, H. influenzae Salmonella
Hyposplenism	Splenectomy; Hemolytic anemia	S. pneumoniae, H. influenzae DF-2

FEVER OF UNKNOWN ORIGIN

A. Definition (Petersdorf RG & Beeson PB, Medicine 40:1,1961)

1) Illness ≥ 3 weeks.
2) Documented fever ≥ 101°F (38.3°C).
3) Negative diagnostic evaluation with 1 week in hospital.

B. Causes (Adapted from: Larson E et al, Medicine 61:269,1982)*

Infections		Neoplastic diseases	33
Abdominal abscesses	32	Lymphoma	6
Mycobacteria	11	Hodgkins	4
Endocarditis	5	Leukemia	5
HIV infection**	0	Lymphomatoid	
Cytomegalovirus	4	granulomatosis	2
Miscellaneous***	12	Malignant histocytosis	4
Collagen disease	8	Pre-leukemia	1
Still's disease	4	Solid tumor****	11
Polyarteritis nodosa	2	Miscellaneous	10
Rheumatic fever	1	Hematoma	3
Polymyalgia rheumatica	0	Pulmonary emboli	1
Rheumatic fever	1	Familial Mediterranean	
Systemic lupus	0	fever	1
Granulomatous disease	9	Myxoma	1
Granulomatous hepatitis	4	Periodic fever	0
Sarcoidosis	2	Factitious fever	3
Giant cell arteritis	1	Undiagnosed	13
Crohn's disease	2		

* This represents an updated version (105 cases; 1970-1980) of the classical report by Petersdorf and Beeson (100 cases, 1952-1957); more recent developments include AIDS and extensive use of scans.

** The Seattle study predated AIDS, but HIV infection would now constitute an important diagnostic consideration.

*** Includes sinusitis, dental infections, osteomyelitis, amebiasis, candidiasis, urinary tract infection.

**** All were solid tumors in the abdomen including hepatoma (2) and hypernephroma (2).

CNS INFECTIONS

I Cerebrospinal Fluid

A. Normal findings

1. Opening pressure: 5-15 mmHg or 65-195 mm H_2O

2. Leukocyte count:<10 mononuclear cells/mm³ (5-10/ml suspect); 1 PMN (5%)

3. Protein: 15-45 mg/dl (higher in elderly)
   Formula: 23.8 × 0.39 × age + 15 mg/100 ml or (more simply) less than patient's age (above 35 yrs).
   Note: WBC's begin to disintegrate after 90 minutes
   Traumatic tap: 1 mg/1000 RBC's

4. Glucose: 40-80 mg% or CSF/blood glucose ratio > 0.6 (with high serum glucose usual ratio is 0.3)

B. Abnormal CSF with non-infectious causes

1. Traumatic tap: Increased protein; RBC's; WBC count and differential proportionate to RBC's in peripheral blood; clear and colorless supernatant of centrifuged CSF.
   Bloody tap: Usually 1 WBC/700 RBC with normal peripheral RBC and WBC counts; if abnormal: true CSF WBC = WBC (CSF) -
   $$\frac{WBC\ (blood) \times RBC\ (CSF)}{RBC\ (blood)}$$

2. Chemical meningitis (injection of anesthetics, chemotherapeutic agents, air, radiographic dyes): Increased protein, lymphocytes (occasionally PMN's).

3. Cerebral contusion, subarachnoid hemorrhage, intracerebral bleed: RBC's, increased protein (1 mg/1000 RBC's), disproportionately increased PMN's (peak at 72-96 hrs); decreased glucose in 15-20%).

4. Vasculitis (SLE, etc): Increased protein (50-100 mg/dl), increased WBC's (usually mononuclear cells, occasionally PMN's); normal glucose.

5. Postictal (repeated generalized seizures): RBC's (0-500/mm³), WBC's (10-100/mm³ with variable % PMN's with peak at 1 day), protein normal or slight increase.

6. Tumors (esp. glioblastomas, leukemia, lymphoma, breast cancer, pancreatic cancer): Low glucose, increased protein, moderate PMN's.

7. Neurosurgery: Blood; increased protein; WBC's (disproportionate to RBC's with predominance of mononuclear cells) up to 2 weeks post-op.

8. Sarcoidosis: Increased protein, WBC's (up to 100/mm³ predominately mononuclear cells); low glucose in 10%.

128

C. <u>CNS infections</u>

	Cell count (/mm^3)	Predominant cell type	Glucose (mg/dl)	Protein (mg/dl)	Microscopic exam	Culture
Meningitis Viral	10-2,000	Monos	40-80	10-45	Neg	Neg
Bacterial Untreated	10-100,000	PMN's	Low	Normal to 600	85-90% pos	90% pos
Partially treated	10-100,000	PMN's	Low or normal	Increased	Variable	Neg, esp with meningococcus or pneumococcus
Tuberculosis	10-1,000	30-100% mono's	Low	Increased 100-500	Rarely pos	Usually positive
Fungal	5-1,000	Mono's	Low or normal	Normal to 500	Rarely pos except India ink prep for Cryptococcus	Usually positive
Encephalitis	0-2,000	Early-PMN's Late-Mono's	Normal	Normal to 120	Neg	Neg
Brain abscess	5-500	Mixed	Normal	Normal to 500	Neg	Neg
AIDS encephalitis/ dementia complex	0-200	Mono's	Normal	Normal to 120	Neg	Often yields HIV

129

II. Meningitis

A. Likely pathogens and treatment

Setting	Likely agent	Empiric treatment* Preferred	Alternative	Comment
Adult, immunocompetent, community-acquired	S. pneumoniae N. meningitidis	Penicillin G	Chloramphenicol Cefotaxime Ceftriaxone Ceftizoxime Ceftazidime Ampicillin	Incresed frequency of Enterobacteriaceae in alcoholics, debilitated and elderly patients: consider third generation cephalosporins for initial treatment
Immunosuppressed Defective humoral immunity, asplenia, complement defect	S. pneumoniae N. meningitidis	As above	As above	
Defective cell-mediated immunity	Listeria Cryptococcus	Ampicillin ± aminoglycoside	Trimethoprim-sulfamethoxazole	Cephalosporins not active vs. Listeria
Post-neurosurgical procedure	Enterobacteriaceae Pseudomonas sp. Staph. aureus	Aminoglycoside + antipseudomonad penicillin (or ceftazidime) + antistaph penicillin (or vancomycin)		In vitro sensitivity tests required, bactericidal activity preferred Infections that are refractory or involve resistant GNB may require intrathecal or intra-ventricular aminoglycosides

Setting	Likely agent	Empiric treatment* Preferred	Empiric treatment* Alternative	Comment
Cranial or spinal trauma Early (0-3 days)	S. pneumoniae	Penicillin or ampicillin	Chloramphenicol	Occasional cases with H. influenzae or Strep. pyogenes
Late (over 3 days)	Enterobacteraceae Pseudomonas S. aureus S. pneumoniae	Treat as recommended for postsurgical complication		
Ventricular shunt	S. epidermidis	Vancomycin	Antistaphylococcal penicillin	In vitro sensitivity tests required Necessity to remove shunt is highly variable; most advocate antibiotics via shunt*

*Antibiotic recommendations assuming clinical ($\pm$ initial CSF analysis) evidence supporting this diagnosis with no direct clues to the etiologic agent.

B. Treatment by organism

Organism	Preferred drug	Alternative	Comment
<u>Strep. pneumoniae</u>	Penicillin G	Chloramphenicol Cefuroxime Cefotaxime Ceftizoxime Ceftriaxone	Test susceptibility to penicillin Resistant strains: chloramphenicol or vancomycin Treat ≥ 10 days
<u>Neisseria meningitidis</u>	Penicillin G	(As above)	Intimate contacts should receive rifampin Treat ≥ 7 days
<u>Haemophilus influenzae</u> Ampicillin sensitive	Ampicillin	Chloramphenicol Cefotaxime Cefuroxime Ceftizoxime Ceftriaxone Ceftazidime	If children< 4 yrs in household, contacts should receive rifampin prophylaxis (type B only) Treat ≥ 10 days
Ampicillin resistant	Chloramphenicol	Cephalosporins (above)	
<u>Listeria monocytogenes</u>	Ampicillin ± aminoglycosides	Trimethoprim-sulfamethoxazole	Cephalosporins are not effective Treat 14-21 days

132

Organism	Preferred drug	Alternative	Comment
E. coli and other coliforms	Cefotaxime Ceftizoxime Ceftriaxone Ceftazidime	Aminoglycoside $\pm$ ampicillin or trimethoprim-sulfamethoxazole	In vitro sensitivity tests required; MBC data preferred Chloramphenicol lacks bactericidal activity vs GNB Aminoglycosides are given systemically $\pm$ intrathecally Treat ≥ 21 days
Pseudomonas aeruginosa	Antipseudomonad penicillin (carbenicillin, ticarcillin, mezlocillin, piperacillin, azlocillin) + aminoglycoside	Aminoglycoside + ceftazidime	Aminoglycoside is given systemically and intrathecally
Staph. aureus	Antistaphylococcal penicillin $\pm$ rifampin	Vancomycin	

III. Doses of Drugs for CNS Infections*

A. Aminoglycosides

Agent	Systemic	Intrathecal/intraventricular
Gentamicin	1.7–2.0 mg/kg (see pg 30,31)	4–5 mg q 12–24 h
Tobramycin	1.7–2.0 mg/kg (see pg 30,31)	4–5 mg q 12–24 h
Amikacin	5.0–7.5 mg/kg (see pg 30,31)	10–12 mg q 12–24 h

B. Cephalosporins

Cefuroxime: 9 gm/day in 3 doses
Cefotaxime: 12 gm/day in 4–6 doses (200 mg/kg q 6 h)**
Ceftizoxime: 12 gm/day in 3–4 doses
Ceftriaxone: 4 gm/day in 2 doses (100 mg/kg q 12 h)**
Ceftazidime: 6 gm/day in 3 doses (125–150 mg/kg q 8 h)**

C. Chloramphenicol: 4–6 gm/day in 4 doses (75–100 mg/kg/day)**

D. Penicillins

Ampicillin: 12 gm/day in 4–6 doses (200–300 mg/kg q 6 h)**

Antipseudomonadal penicillins
    Ticarcillin: 18–24 gm/day in 6 doses (40–60 mg/kg q 4 h)
    Mezlocillin: 18–24 gm/day in 6 doses (40–60 mg/kg q 4 h)
    Azlocillin: 18–24 gm/day in 6 doses (40–60 mg/kg q 4 h)
    Piperacillin: 18–24 gm/day in 6 doses (40–60 mg/kg q 4 h)

Antistaphylococcal penicillins
    Nafcillin: 9–12 gm/day in 6 doses (20–30 mg/kg q 4 h)
    Oxacillin: 9–12 gm/day in 6 doses (20–30 mg/kg q 4 h)
    Methicillin: 9–12 gm/day in 6 doses (20–30 mg/kg q 4 h)

Penicillin G: 18 million units/day in 6 doses (250,000 U/kg/day)**

E. Trimethoprim-sulfamethoxazole: 15–20 mg/kg/day (trimethoprim) in 4 doses
Metronidazole: 2 gm/day in 2–4 doses
Vancomycin: 2 gm/day in 2–4 doses (40–60 mg/kg/day)**

* Assume adult patient with normal renal function.
** Recommendation of American Academy of Pediatrics (Pediatrics 78(Suppl)959, 1986).

C. Aseptic Meningitis: Infectious and Non-infectious Causes* (from American Academy of Pediatrics, Pediatrics 78 (Supplement):970,1986)

Infectious Agents and Diseases
Bacteria: Partially treated meningitis, Mycobacterium tuberculosis, parameningeal focus (brain abscess, epidural abscess), acute or subacute bacterial endocarditis
Viruses: Enteroviruses, mumps, lymphocytic choriomeningitis, Epstein-Barr, arboviruses (Eastern equine, Western equine, St Louis), cytomegalovirus, varicella-zoster, herpes simplex, human immunodeficiency virus
Ricketsiae: Rocky Mountain spotted fever
Spirochetes: Syphilis, leptospirosis, Lyme disease
Mycoplasma: M pneumoniae, M hominis (neonates)
Fungi: Candida albicans, Coccidioides immitis, Cryptococcus neoformans
Protozoa: Toxoplasma gondii, malaria, amoebas, visceral larval migrans (Taenia canis)
Nematode: Rat lung worm larvae (eosinophilic meningitis)
Cestodes: Cysticercosis
Non-infectious Diseases
Malignancy: Primary medulloblastoma, metastatic leukemia, Hodgkin disease
Collagen-vascular disease: Lupus erythematosus
Trauma: Subarachnoid bleed, traumatic lumbar puncture, neurosurgery
Granulomatous disease: Sarcoidosis
Direct toxin: Intrathecal injections of contrast media, spinal anesthesia
Poison: Lead, mercury
Autoimmune disease: Guillain-Barre syndrome
Unknown: Multiple sclerosis, Mollaret's meningitis, Behcet syndrome, Vogt-Koyanagi syndrome, Harada syndrome, Kawasaki disease

* Aseptic meningitis is defined as meningitis in the absence of evidence of a bacterial pathogen detectable in CSF by usual laboratory techniques.

UPPER RESPIRATORY TRACT INFECTIONS

Condition	Usual Pathogens	Preferred Treatment	Alternatives	Comment
Ear & Mastoids				
Acute otitis media	S. pneumoniae H. influenzae	Ampicillin or amoxicillin Erythromycin	Trimethoprim-sulfamethoxazole Cefaclor Amoxicillin + clavulinate	Tympanocentesis rarely indicated Less frequent pathogens: S. aureus, Strep. pyogenes, Moraxella catarrhalis
Chronic suppurative otitis media	Pseudomonas Staphylococci Proteus, E. coli B. fragilis	Neomycin/ polymyxin otic drops	Chloramphenicol otic drops	
Malignant otitis externa	P. aeruginosa	Tobramycin or amikacin + ticarcillin, mezlocillin or pipericillin	Tobramycin or amikacin + cefoperazone, ceftazidime, imipenem or ciprofloxacin	Surgical drainage and/or debridement sometimes required
Acute diffuse otitis media ("swimmers ear")	P. aeruginosa Coliforms Staph. aureus	Neomycin/ polymyxin otic drops	Boric or acetic acid (2%) drops	
Otomycosis	Aspergillus niger	Boric or acetic acid drops	M-cresyl acetic otic drops	
Acute mastoiditis	S. pneumoniae H. influenzae	Cefuroxime or trimethoprim- sulfamethoxazole	Amoxicillin or ampicillin Amoxicillin + clavulinate	Surgery often required

136

Condition	Usual Pathogens	Preferred Treatment	Alternatives	Comment
Chronic mastoiditis	Anaerobes Pseudomonas sp Coliforms	None		Surgery often required
Sinusitis Acute sinusitis	H. influenzae S. pneumoniae	Amoxicillin or ampicillin	Trimethoprim-sulfamethoxazole Cefaclor, cefuroxime Amoxicillin + clavulinate Erythromycin	Nasal decongestant Alternative regimens are active vs. most amp-resistant strains of H. influenzae
Chronic sinusitis	Anaerobes S. aureus	Penicillin or ampicillin Clindamycin (if septic)	Amoxicillin + clavulinate	Reserve antibiotic treatment for acute flares
Nosocomial sinusitis	Pseudomonas Coliforms	Aminoglycoside + anti-pseudomonad penicillin or Aminoglycoside + cephalosporin	Imipenem, cephalosporin - 3rd generation	Complication of nasal intubation
Pharynx Pharyngitis	Strep. pyogenes Corynebacterium hemolyticum (mycoplasma, viruses including EBV)	Penicillin (strep only)	Erythromycin	If compliance questionable use benzathine pen G x 1 IM; treatment with oral pen V or erythromycin for 10 days
Gonococcal pharyngitis	N. gonorrhoeae	Ceftriaxone	Aq procaine penicillin + probenecid, trimethoprim-sulfa	Most cases are asymptomatic

Condition	Usual Pathogens	Preferred Treatment	Alternatives	Comment
Peritonsillar or tonsillar abscess	Strep. pyogenes Peptostreptococci	Penicillin G	Clindamycin	Drainage necessary
Membranous pharyngitis	C. diphtheriae Epstein-Barr virus Vincent's angina (anaerobes)	Penicillin or erythromycin (diphtheria) Penicillin (anaerobes)		Diphtheria: Antitoxin
Epiglottitis	H. influenzae	Chloramphenicol ± ampicillin	Cefuroxime, cefamandole, cefotaxime, ceftizoxime, ceftriaxone, ceftazidime	Ensure patent airway If isolate of H. influenzae in patient treated with chloro is amp-sensitive change to ampicillin
Laryngitis	Viruses (M. catarrhalis)			For M. catarrhalis: trimethoprim-sulfa, erythromycin or amoxicillin-clavulinate, cefaclor
Perimandibular Actinomycosis	A. israelii	Penicillin G or V	Clindamycin, tetracycline, erythromycin	Treat for 3-6 months
Parotitis	S. aureus (anaerobes)	Penicillinase-resistant penicillin	Cephalosporin (1st generation) Clindamycin, vancomycin	
Space infections	Anaerobes	Penicillin Clindamycin	Cefoxitin, penicillin + metronidazole	Drainage necessary

Condition	Usual Pathogens	Preferred Treatment	Alternatives	Comment
Cervical				
Cervical adenitis acute	S. aureus Strep. pyogenes Anaerobes Viral Toxoplasmosis	Penicillin (S. pyogenes, anaerobes) Penicillinase- resistant penicillin (S. aureus)	Erythromycin Clindamycin Amoxicillin + clavulinate (Bacterial infections)	
Cervical adenitis chronic	Mycobacteria, Cat scratch disease HIV infection			Non-infectious causes include tumors, lymphoma, sarcoid
Dental				
Periapical abscess Gum boil Gingivitis Pyorrhoea	Anaerobes Streptococci	Penicillin Clindamycin	Metronidazole + penicillin	Metronidazole often preferred for periodontal disease, e.g. gingivitis, periodontitis
Stomatitis				
Thrush	C. albicans	Oral nystatin or clotrimazole	Ketoconazole po	
Vincent's angina	Anaerobes	Penicillin Clindamycin	Metronidazole, tetracycline	
Aphthous stomatitis	No pathogen identified			
Herpetiform ulcers	H. simplex	Acyclovir		Usually reserved for immunocompromised hosts

139

Cost of Oral Drugs Commonly Used for Upper Respiratory Infections

	Wholesale price for 10 day supply*
Penicillins	
Penicillin G: 400,000 units po qid	$ 2.40** ($5.00)
Penicillin V: 500 mg po qid	$ 3.20** ($9.20)
Ampicillin: 500 mg po qid	$ 6.00** ($13.00)
Amoxicillin: 250 mg po tid	$ 5.00** ($6.30)
Amoxicillin + clavulinate 250 mg po tid	$31.00
Dicloxacillin: 500 mg po qid	$23.00** ($70.00)
Cephalosporins	
Cefaclor: 250 mg po qid	$48.00 -
Cephalexin: 250 mg po qid	$14.00** ($30.00)
Cephradine: 250 mg po qid	$18.00** ($30.00)
Cefuroxime axetil: 250 mg po bid	$36.00 -
Clindamycin: 300 mg po tid	$55.00 -
Trimethoprim-sulfamethoxazole: 1 DS bid	$ 3.80** ($12.80)
Metronidazole: 500 mg po bid	$ 2.80** ($28.00)
Erythromycin: 500 mg po qid	$10.00** ($17.60)
Tetracycline: 500 mg po qid	$ 2.40** ($5.20)
Doxycycline: 100 mg po bid	$ 4.00** ($41.00)

* Approximate wholesale prices according to "American Druggist Blue Book 1988-1989. (Prices to patient will be higher).

** Price provided is for generic product; price in parentheses is for a representative brand product.

140

PULMONARY INFECTIONS

A. **Specimens and Tests for Detection of Lower Respiratory Pathogens**
(Reprinted with permission from: Bartlett JG et al: Cumitech 7A, Sept 1987, pg 3)

Organism	Specimen	Microscopy	Culture	Serology	Other
Bacteria					
Aerobic and facultatively anaerobic	Expectorated sputum, blood, TTA, empyema fluid, lung biopsy	Gram stain	X		
Anaerobic	TTA, empyema fluid, tissue, abscess	Gram stain	X		
Legionella sp.	Sputum, lung biopsy, pleural fluid, TTA, serum	FA	X	FA	
Nocardia sp.	Expectorated sputum, TTA, bronchial washings, BAL fluid, tissue, abscess	Gram and/or modified carbol fuchsin stain	X		
Chlamydia sp.	Nasopharyngeal swab, lung aspirate or biopsy, serum		X	FA for *C. trachomatis* and CF for *C. psittaci*	
Mycoplasma sp.	Expectorated sputum, nasopharyngeal swab, serum		X	CF, FA, or MI; cold agglutinins	
Mycobacteria	Expectorated or induced sputum, bronchial washings, BAL fluid, tissue, gastric washings	Fluorochrome stain or carbol fuchsin	X		PPD
Fungi					
Deep-seated					
Blastomyces sp.	Expectorated or induced sputum, TTA, bronchial washing or biopsy, BAL fluid, tissue, serum	KOH with phase contrast; GMS stain	X	CF, ID	
Coccidioides sp.				CF, ID, LA	
Histoplasma sp.				CF, ID	
Opportunistic					
Aspergillus sp.	Lung biopsy, serum	H & E, GMS stain	X	ID	
Candida sp.	Lung biopsy, serum	H & E, GMS stain	X	ID, CIE, LA	
Cryptococcus sp.	Expectorated sputum, serum	H & E, GMS stain, Calcofluor white	X	LA	
Zygomycetes	Expectorated sputum, tissue	H & E, GMS stain	X		
Viruses	Nasal washings, nasopharyngeal aspirate or swab, BAL fluid, lung biopsy, serum	FA	X	CF, EIA, LA, FA	
Pneumocystis sp.	Lung biopsy, TTA, bronchial brushings or washings, BAL fluid	Toluidine blue, Giemsa, or GMS stain			

[a] Abbreviations: CF, complement fixation; MI, metabolic inhibition; PPD, purified protein derivative; ID, immunodiffusion; LA, latex agglutination; H & E, hematoxylin and eosin; CIE, counterimmunoelectrophoresis; EIA, enzyme immunoassay.

141

B. Preferred Antibiotics for Pulmonary Infections

Agent	Preferred antimicrobial	Alternatives	Comment
Bacteria			
S. pneumoniae	Penicillin G or V	Ampicillin/amoxicillin Cephalosporins Erythromycin Clindamycin Tetracycline Chloramphenicol	Most quinolones (ciprofloxacin) and aminoglycosides are inactive in vitro; some 3rd generation cephalosporins (ceftriaxone) are relatively inactive
Enterobacteriaceae (coliforms)	Aminoglycoside + cephalosporin, antipseudomonad penicillin, or imipenem	Cephalosporin (alone) Ciprofloxacin ± aminoglycoside Aztreonam ± second agent Sulfa-trimethoprim	In vitro sensitivity tests required
Pseudomonas aeruginosa	Aminoglycoside + antipseudomonad penicillin, ceftazidime or imipenem	Ciprofloxacin ± aminoglycoside	In vitro sensitivity tests required Antimicrobial combinations required for serious infections
Moraxella catarrhalis (Branhamella catarrhalis)	Trimethoprim-sulfa Erythromycin	Tetracycline Amoxicillin + clavulanic acid Cephalosporins	70-80% of strains produce betalactamase

Agent	Preferred antimicrobial	Alternatives	Comment
S. aureus Methicillin-sens	Penicillinase resistant penicillin (nafcillin, oxacillin)	Cephalosporin - 1st generation or cefamandole/cefuroxime Vancomycin Clindamycin	May add aminoglycoside or rifampin for serious or refractory infections
Methicillin-resist	Vancomycin	Ciprofloxacin Sulfa-trimethoprim	
H. influenzae	Ampicillin/amoxicillin Cefamandole/cefuroxime Sulfa-trimethoprim	Cephalosporins - 3rd generation Tetracycline Chloramphenicol	15-30% of strains are ampicillin resistant
Anaerobes	Clindamycin	Penicillin Metronidazole + penicillin	Penicillins other than anti-staphylococcal agents are equally effective compared to penicillin G Cephalosporins (esp cefoxitin) are probably effective, but published experience is limited Metronidazole should not be used alone
Mycoplasma	Tetracycline Erythromycin		Treat for 1-2 weeks
TWAR	Tetracycline	Erythromycin	Treat for 10-21 days

Agent	Preferred antimicrobial	Alternatives	Comment
Legionella	Erythromycin	Erythromycin + rifampin Sulfa-trimethoprim + rifampin	Treat for 3 weeks
Nocardia	Sulfonamide	Doxycycline Sulfa-trimethoprim	Usual sulfa is sulfadiazine Treat 3-6 months
Mycobacteria M. tuberculosis	INH plus rifampin ± pyrazinamide		See pg 96-99
M. avium	INH, ethambutol rifampin and streptomycin	Additional agents: Ethionamide, ansamycin cycloserine, ciprofloxacin, kanamycin, amikacin clofazimine, enviomycin	Recommended regimen is for moderately advanced pulmonary disease; 5-6 drugs advocated for far advanced disease or progression during treatment; no regimen has established efficacy in AIDS Treat for 2 years
M. kansasii	INH, rifampin, and ethambutol		Treat for 18 months

Agent	Preferred antimicrobial	Alternatives	Comment
Fungi			See pg 79-86
Aspergillus	Amphotericin B		
Blastomyces	Ketoconazole	Amphotericin B	
Coccidioides	Ketoconazole	Amphotericin B	
Cryptococcus	Amphotericin B $\pm$ fluconazole	Ketoconazole	
Histoplasma	Ketoconazole	Amphotericin B	
Phycomycetes (mucor)	Amphotericin B		
Viruses			See pg 91-95
Influenza A	Amantidine		
Herpes simplex	Acyclovir		
Varicella-zoster	Acyclovir		
Cytomegalovirus	Ganciclovir (investigational)		Efficacy in CMV pneumonitis is not clearly established
Parasites			See pg 120,121
Pneumocystis carinii	Sulfa-trimethoprim	Pentamidine Trimetrexate (investigational) Dapsone + Trimethoprim	

TREATMENT OF ENDOCARDITIS

(Committee on Rheumatic Fever, Endocarditis and Kawasaki Disease of the American Heart Association's Council on Cardiovascular Disease in the Young: Antimicrobial Treatment of Infective Endocarditis due to Viridans Streptococci, Enterococci and Staphylococci and Staphylococci. JAMA 261:1471,1989)

I

A. Medical Management

A. Penicillin sensitive streptococci (minimum inhibitory concentration < 0.1 µg/mL)

A. Streptococci

1. **Penicillin only:** Aqueous penicillin G, 10-20 million units/day IV x 4 weeks. (Preferred regimen for patients with a relative contraindication to streptomycin including age > 65 years, renal impairment or prior 8th cranial nerve damage.)

2. **Penicillin + streptomycin x 4 weeks:** Aqueous penicillin G, 1.2 million units IM q 6 h or aqueous penicillin G, 10-20 million units/day IV x 4 weeks plus streptomycin, 7.5 mg/kg IM (up to 500 mg) q 12 h or gentamicin, 1 mg/kg IM or IV (up to 80 mg) q 8 h for first 2 weeks. (The disadvantage of the procaine penicillin + streptomycin is the necessity of 140 IM injections.)

3. **Two week course:** Procaine penicillin G, 1.2 million units q 6 h IM or aqueous penicillin G, 10-20 million units/day IV x 4 weeks plus streptomycin, 7.5 mg/kg IM (up to 500 mg) q 12 h or gentamicin, 1 mg/kg IM or IV q 8 h x 4 wks in 2-4 doses. (Advocated as most cost-effective regimen by Mayo Clinic group for uncomplicated cases with relapse rates of < 1%.)

4. **Penicillin allergy:** Vancomycin, 30 mg/kg/day IV x 4 weeks in 2-4 doses not to exceed 2 gm/day unless serum levels are monitored.

5. **Penicillin allergy, cephalosporins:** Cephalothin, 2 gm q 4 h x 4 wks or cefazolin, 1 gm IM or IV q 8 h x 4 wks. (Avoid in patients with immediate hypersensitivity to penicillin.)

Note

1. Aqueous penicillin G should be given in 6 equally divided daily doses or by continuous infusion; disadvantage of procaine penicillin is the large number of IM injections.

2. Streptococcus bovis and tolerant streptococci with MIC < 0.1 µg/mL may receive any of these regimens.

3. Nutritionally deficient streptococci with MIC < 0.1 µg/mL should receive regimen #2 with IV penicillin; if susceptibility cannot be reliably determined treat for MIC > 0.1 mg/mL and < 0.5 µg/mL.

4. Prosthetic valve endocarditis: Regimen #2 with IV penicillin for 6 weeks and aminoglycoside (streptomycin or gentamicin) for at least two weeks.

5. Streptococci with MIC's > 1000 mg/mL to streptomycin should be treated with gentamicin in aminoglycoside containing regimens. Gentamicin and streptomycin are considered equally effective for strains sensitive to both. An advantage of gentamicin is the ability to administer IV as well as IM.

6. Cephalosporin regimens: Other cephalosporins may be effective, but clinical experience for agents other than cephalothin and cefazolin is limited.

7. Two week treatment regimen is not recommended for complicated cases, e.g. shock, extracardiac foci of infection or intracardiac abscess.

8. Desired peak serum levels if obtained: Streptomycin - 20 μg/mL, gentamicin - 3 μg/mL, vancomycin - 20-35 μg/mL (qid), or 30-45 μg/mL (bid).

B. Viridans streptococci and Streptococcus bovis relatively resistant to penicillin G (minimum inhibitory concentration > 0.1 μg/mL and < 0.5 μg/mL).

1. Aqueous penicillin G, 20 million units/day IV x 4 weeks plus streptomycin, 7.5 mg/kg IM (up to 500 mg) q 12 h or gentamicin, 1.0 mg/kg (up to 80 mg) q 8 h x 2 wks.

2. Penicillin allergy: Vancomycin, 30 mg/kg/day x 4 wks in 2-4 daily doses.

3. Penicillin allergy, cephalosporins: Cephalothin, 2 gm IV q 4 h or cefazolin, 1 gm IM or IV q 8 h x 4 wks.

C. Penicillin resistant streptococci including enterococci and strains with minimum inhibitory concentrations of > 0.5 μg/ml.

1. Penicillin + aminoglycoside:
   Aqueous penicillin G   Streptomycin, 7.5 mg/kg IM q 12 h } 4-6
   20-30 million units/day IV plus   or   wks
                              Gentamicin, 1 mg/kg IM or IV q 8 h
   Ampicillin, 12 mg/day IV

2. Penicillin allergy: Vancomycin + aminoglycoside
   Vancomycin, 30 mg/kg/day plus Streptomycin, 7.5 mg/kg IM q 12 h } 4-6
   IV in 2-4 doses   or   wks
                              Gentamicin 1 mg/kg IM or IV q 8 h

Note

1. Choice of aminoglycoside is usually determined by in vitro sensitivity testing. Gentamicin and streptomycin are considered equally effective for treatment of strains susceptible at 2000 μg/mL; high level resistance is more likely with streptomycin so that gentamicin is preferred when in vitro testing cannot be done. Other aminoglycosides should not be used.

2. Occasional strains produce beta-lactamase and should be treated with vancomycin.

3. Patients with symptoms for over 3 months prior to treatment and those with prosthetic valve endocarditis should receive combined treatment for 6 wks.

4. Serum levels of aminoglycosides should be monitored. Desirable peak levels are: Streptomycin - 20 μg/mL and gentamicin - 3 μg/mL.

II Staphylococcus aureus or S. epidermidis

A. No prosthetic device - methicillin sensitive

1. Nafcillin or oxacillin, 2 gm IV q 4 h x 4-6 wks ± gentamicin, 1 mg/kg IV or IM q 8 h x 3-5 days.

2. Penicillin allergy, cephalosporin: Cephalothin, 2 gm IV q 4 h or cefazolin, 2 gm IV q 8 h x 4-6 wks ± gentamicin, 1 mg/kg IV or IM q 8 h x 3-5 days (should not be used with immediate type penicillin hypersensitivity).

3. Penicillin allergy: Vancomycin, 30 mg/kg/day in 2-4 doses (not to exceed 2 gm/day unless serum levels monitored) x 4-6 wks.

4. Methicillin resistant strain: Vancomycin, 30 mg/kg/day in 2-4 doses (not to exceed 2 gm/day unless serum levels monitored) x 4-6 wks.

B. Prosthetic valve or prosthetic material

1. Methicillin-sensitive strains: Nafcillin, 2 gm IV q 4 h x ≥ 6 wks plus rifampin, 300 mg po q 8 h x ≥ 6 wks plus gentamicin, 1 mg/kg IV or IM (not to exceed 80 mg) x 2 wks.

2. Methicillin-resistant strains: Vancomycin, 30 mg/kg/day (not to exceed 2 gm/day unless serum levels monitored) x ≥ 6 wks plus rifampin, 300 mg po q 8 h x ≥ 6 wks plus gentamicin, 1 mg/kg IV or IM (not to exceed 80 mg) x 2 wks.

Note

1. Methicillin resistant staphylococci should be considered resistant to cephalosporins.

2. Tolerance has no important effect on antibiotic selection.

3. The occasional strains of staphylococci that are sensitive to penicillin G at ≤ 0.1 μg/mL may be treated with regimens advocated for penicillin-sensitive streptococci.

4. For native valve endocarditis, the addition of gentamicin to nafcillin or oxacillin causes a more rapid clearing of bacteremia, but has no impact on cure rates; use of gentamicin (or rifampin) with either methicillin-sensitive or methicillin-resistant strains is arbitrary. With vancomycin regimens, there is evidence for synergistic nephrotoxic effects and no enhanced efficacy; addition of aminoglycosides should be restricted to cases involving aminoglycoside-sensitive strains and duration limited to 3-5 days.

5. Coagulase-negative strains infecting prosthetic valves should be considered methicillin-resistant unless sensitivity is conclusively demonstrated.

6. Aminoglycoside selection for coagulase negative strains should be selected on basis of in vitro sensitivity tests; if not active, these agents should be omitted.

B. Indications for Cardiac Surgery in Patients with Endocarditis (Alsip SG, et al: Amer J Med 78(suppl 6B):138,1985)

I. Indications for urgent cardiac surgery

Hemodynamic compromise
   Severe heart failure (esp with aortic insufficiency)
   Vascular obstruction
Uncontrolled infection
   Fungal endocarditis
   Persistent bacteremia (or persistent signs of sepsis)
   Lack of effective antimicrobial agents
Unstable prosthetic valve

II. Relative indications for cardiac surgery

1. Native valve
   Bacterial agent other than susceptible streptococci
      (such as S. aureus or gram neg bacilli)
   Relapse (esp if non-streptococcal agent)
   Evidence of intracardiac extension
      Rupture of sinus of Valsalva or ventricular septum
      Ruptured chordae tendineae or papillary muscle
      Heart block (new conduction disturbance)
      Abscess shown by echo or catheterization
   Two or more emboli
   Vegetations demonstrated by echo (especially large
      vegetation or aortic valve vegetations)
   Mitral valve preclosure by echo (correlates with severe acute
      aortic insufficiency)

2. Prosthetic valve
   Early post-operative endocarditis (< 8 wks)
   Nonstreptococcal late endocarditis
   Periprosthetic leak
   Two or more emboli
   Relapse
   Evidence of intracardiac extension (see above)
   Miscellaneous: Heart failure, aortic valve involvement, new
      or increased regurgitant murmur or mechanical valve
      versus bioprosthesis

III. Point system: Urgent surgery should be strongly considered with 5
   accumulated points (Cobbs CG and Gnann JW: Indications for surgery
   in infective endocarditis. In Sande MA, Kaye D (Eds) Contemporary
   Issues in Infectious Disease. Churchill Livingstone, New York, 1984,
   pp 201-212)

	Native valve	Prosthetic valve
Heart failure		
Severe	5	5
Moderate	3	5
Mild	1	2
Fungal etiology	5	5
Persistent bacteremia	5	5
Organism other than susceptible strep	1	2
Relapse	2	3
One major embolus	2	2
Two or more systemic emboli	4	4
Vegetations by echocardiography	1	1
Ruptured chordae tendinae or papillary mm.	3	-
Ruptured sinus of Valsalva	4	4
Ruptured ventricular septum	4	4
Heart block	3	3
Early mitral valve closure by echo	2	-
Unstable prosthesis	-	5
Early prosthetic valve endocarditis	-	2
Periprosthetic leak	-	2

INTRA-ABDOMINAL SEPSIS: ANTIBIOTIC SELECTION

1. **Peritonitis**

   A. _Polymicrobial infection_

   1. Combination treatment*

      An aminoglycoside vs. coliforms

      a. Gentamicin, 2.0 mg/kg, then 1.7 mg/kg IV q 8 h (usually preferred) _or_
      b. Tobramycin, 2.0 mg/kg, then 1.7 mg/kg IV q 8 h _or_
      c. Amikacin, 7.5 mg/kg, then 5.0 mg/kg IV q 8 h

      Plus an agent vs. anaerobes

      a. Clindamycin, 600 mg IV q 8 h _or_
      b. Cefoxitin, 2 gm IV q 6 h _or_
      c. Metronidazole, 500 mg IV q 8 h

      ---

      * Some authorities add an agent for the enterococcus:
        Ampicillin, 1-2 gm IV q 6 h

   2. Single drug treatment

      a. Cefoxitin, 2 gm IV q 6 h (Not advocated as single agent if infection acquired during hospitalization or if there has been antibiotic administration during prior two weeks)

      b. Imipenem, 500 mg IV q 6-8 h

      c. Ticarcillin, 3 gm + clavulanic acid, 100 mg (Timentin) IV q 4-6 h

      d. Ampicillin, 2 gm + sulbactam, 1 gm (Unasyn) IV q 6 h

   B. _Monomicrobial infections_

   1. Spontaneous peritonitis or "primary peritonitis"

      a. Gentamicin or tobramycin, 2 mg/kg IV, then 1.7 mg/kg IV q 8 h _plus_ a betalactam: Cefazolin, 2 gm IV q 8 h; cefoxitin, 2 gm IV q 6 h; cefotaxime, 1.5-2 gm IV q 6 h; ampicillin, 2 gm IV q 6 h; or piperacillin, 4-5 gm IV q 6 h

      b. Cefotaxime, 1.5-2 gm IV q 6 h ± ampicillin, 2 gm IV q 6 h

   2. Peritonitis associated with peritoneal dialysis

      a. Vancomycin, 1 gm IV (single dose)

b. Antibiotics added to dialysate based on in vitro sensitivity: Nafcillin, 10 mg/L; ampicillin, 20 mg/L; ticarcillin, 100 mg/L; penicillin G, 1,000-2,000 units/L; cephalothin, 20 mg/L; gentamicin or tobramycin, 5 mg/L; amikacin, 25 mg/L; clindamycin, 10 mg/L

3. Candida peritonitis

a. Amphotericin B, 200-1000 mg (total dose) 1 mg IV over 6 hrs, then increase by 5-10 mg/day to maintenance dose of 20-30 mg/day

b. Peritoneal dialysis: Systemic amphotericin B (above regimen) plus addition to dialysate, 2-5 μg/ml

4. Tuberculous
INH, 300 mg/day po, plus rifampin, 600 mg/day po, plus pyrazinamide, 15-30 mg/kg/day po x 2 months, then INH plus rifampin x 7-22 months

II Localized Infections

A. Intra-abdominal abscess(es) (not further defined): Use regimens recommended for polymicrobial infections with peritonitis.

B. Liver abscess

1. Amebic

a. Preferred: Metronidazole, 750 mg po tid x 20 days plus iodoquinol, 650 mg po tid x 20 days

b. Alternative: Emetine, 1-1.5 mg/kg/day IM x 5 days (or dehydro-emetine, 1-1.5 mg/kg/day x 5 days) followed by chloroquine, 500 mg po bid x 2 days, then 250 mg po bid x 3 weeks plus iodoquinol, 650 mg po tid x 20 days

2. Pyogenic

a. Gentamicin or tobramycin, 2.0 mg/kg IV, then 1.7 mg/kg IV q 8 h plus metronidazole, 500 mg IV q 8 h; clindamycin, 600 mg IV q 8 h, or cefoxitin, 2 gm IV q 6 h plus ampicillin, 2 gm IV q 6 h or penicillin G, 2 million units IV q 6 h

b. Gentamicin or tobramycin (above doses) plus clindamycin (above doses), cefoxitin (above doses) or piperacillin 4-5 gm IV q 6 h

C. Biliary tract infections

1. Cholecystitis

a. Combination treatment: Gentamicin or tobramycin, 2.0 mg/kg IV, then 1.7 mg/kg IV q 8 h plus ampicillin, 2 gm IV q 6 h, piperacillin, 2-5 gm IV q 6 h, or cefoperazone, 1-2 gm IV q 12 h*

b. Single agent: Cefoperazone, 1-2 gm IV q 12 h*

* Other cephalosporins (2nd and 3rd generation) are probably equally effective. Some authorities add ampicillin (1-2 gm IV q 6 h) to cephalosporin containing regimens

2. Ascending cholangitis, empyema of the gall bladder, or emphasematous cholecystitis: Treat with regimens advocated for peritonitis or intra-abdominal abscess

D. Appendicitis (adult doses)*

1. Combination treatment: Gentamicin or tobramycin, 2.0 mg/kg IV, then 1.7 mg/kg q 8 h plus clindamycin, 600 mg IV q 8 h, cefoxitin, 2 gm IV q 6 h or metronidazole, 500 mg IV q 6 h

2. Single agent: Cefoxitin, 2 gm IV q 6 h

* Role of antibiotics in nonperforative appendicitis is unclear.

E. Diverticulitis*

1. Ambulatory patient

   a. Ampicillin, 500 mg po qid
   b. Tetracycline, 500 mg po qid
   c. Amoxicillin plus clavulanic acid (Augmentin), 500 mg po qid
   d. Cephalexin, 500 mg po qid plus metronidazole, 500 mg po qid

2. Hospitalized patients: Use regimens advocated for peritonitis or intra-abdominal abscess

* Role of antibiotics in uncomplicated diverticulitis is unclear

153

HEPATITIS

A. Types, clinical features and prognosis (MMWR 34:313,1985 and MMWR 37:341,1988)

Type	Source	Incubation period	Diagnosis of acute viral hepatitis*	Prognosis
A (HAV)	Person-to-person fecal-oral Contaminated food & water (epidemic)	15-50 days Avg: 28 days	IgM-anti HAV (see serologic events)	Self limited: >99% Fulminant & fatal: 0.6% No carrier state Severity increases with age
B (HBV)	Sexual contact or contaminated needles from HBsAg carrier source (Transmission via blood transfusions is rare due to HBsAg screening) Efficacy of transmission increased if source is HBeAg positive Needle stick injury with HBsAg carrier source: 6-30% transmission Perinatal with HBsAg carrier mother: 70-90% transmission	45-160 days Avg: 60-120 days	HBsAg and/or IgM anti HBc	Fulminant & fatal:<2% Carrier state: 6-10% Chronic hepatitis: 25% of carriers with 15-30% developing cirrhosis Perinatal transmission: Chronic carrier in 85-90%, of whom 25% progress to fatality due to cirrhosis or hepatocellular carcinoma

154

Type	Source	Incubation period	Diagnosis of acute viral hepatitis*	Prognosis
(HCV) (NANB) post-transfusion	Contaminated blood and needles (U.S. and Europe)	14-84 days	Neg IgM anti HAV and neg HBsAg and/or IgM anti-HBc	Fulminant & fatal: rare Chronic carriers: 50%
E (HEV) enterally transmitted	Epidemic fecal-oral (Southeast Asia, North Africa, India, Soviet Union, Mexico)	30-50 days	As above	Mortality in pregnant women is 10-20% for enterally transmitted NANB
Delta	Defective virus that requires presence of active HBV, e.g. co-infection with HBV or superinfection in HBsAg carrier; main source is blood (IV drug abuse, hemophilia)	Superinfection: 30-60 days Co-infection: same as HBV	ABsAg + anti-HDV limited availability Acute: Appears late and short-lived Co-infection: IgM anti-HBc + anti-HDV Chronic: Persistent HBs + anti-HDV in high titer	Co-infection with HBV: 1-10% acute fatality; <5% chronic hepatitis Superinfection: 5-20% acute fatality; >75% chronic hepatitis with 70-80% developing cirrhosis

* Symptoms or signs of viral hepatitis, serum aminotransferase > 2.5 x upper limit of normal, and absence of other causes of liver injury.

B. Hepatitis nomenclature

Abbreviation	Term	Comments
Hepatitis A		
HAV	Hepatitis A virus	Etiologic agent of "infectious" hepatitis; a picornavirus; single serotype.
Anti-HAV	Antibody to HAV	Detectable at onset of symptoms; lifetime persistence.
IgM anti-HAV	IgM class antibody to HAV	Indicates recent infection with hepatitis A; positive up to 4–6 months after infection.
Hepatitis B		
HBV	Hepatitis B virus	Etiologic agent of "serum" or "long-incubation" hepatitis; also known as Dane particle.
HBsAg	Hepatitis B surface antigen	Surface antigen(s) of HBV detectable in large quantity in serum; several subtypes identified.
HBeAg	Hepatitis B e antigen	Soluble antigen; correlates with HBV replication, high titer HBV in serum, and infectivity of serum.
HBcAg	Hepatitis B core antigen	No commercial test available.
Anti-HBs	Antibody to HBsAg	Indicates past infection with and immunity to HBV, passive antibody from HBIG, or immune response from HBV vaccine.
Anti-HBe	Antibody to HBeAg	Presence in serum of HBsAg carrier suggests lower titer of HBV.
Anti-HBc	Antibody to HBcAg	Indicates past infection with HBV at some undefined time.
IgM anti-HBc	IgM class antibody to HBcAg	Indicates recent infection with HBV; positive for 4–6 months after infection.
Delta hepatitis		
δ virus	Delta virus	Etiologic agent of delta hepatitis; may only cause infection in presence of HBV.
δ-Ag	Delta antigen	Detectable in early acute delta infection.
Anti-δ	Antibody to delta antigen	Indicates past or present infection with delta virus.
Non-A, non-B		
NANB	Non-A, non-B hepatitis	Diagnosis of exclusion. At least two candidate viruses; epidemiology parallels that of hepatitis B.
Epidemic non-A, non-B hepatitis		
Epidemic NANB	Epidemic non-A, non-B hepatitis	Causes large epidemics in Asia, North Africa; fecal-oral or waterborne.
Immune globulins		
IG	Immune globulin (previously ISG, immune serum globulin, or gamma globulin)	Contains antibodies to HAV, low titer antibodies to HBV.
HBIG	Hepatitis B immune globulin	Contains high titer antibodies to HBV.

C. Hepatitis serologic events for HAV and HBV

1. HAV

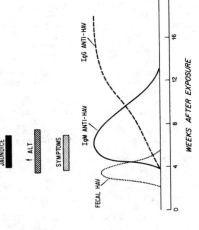

WEEKS AFTER EXPOSURE

JAUNDICE
↑ ALT
SYMPTOMS

IgG ANTI-HAV

IgM ANTI-HAV

FECAL HAV

2. HBV

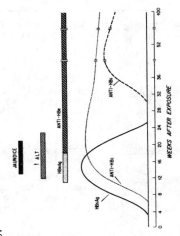

WEEKS AFTER EXPOSURE

JAUNDICE
↑ ALT
HBsAg
ANTI-HBe

ANTI-HBs

ANTI-HBc

HBsAg

D. Hepatitis vaccine recommendations: See page 65-67.
   Note: Revised recommendation by ACIP is for routine HBsAg testing of all pregnant women during an early prenatal visit in each pregnancy; if HBsAg positive the newborn should receive HBIG and HB vaccine at birth (MMWR 37:341,1988).

157

A. Antimicrobial Treatment

Agent	Preferred	Alternative	Comment
Bacteria			
Aeromonas hydrophilia	Sulfa-trimethoprim 1 DS bid x 5 days	Ciprofloxacin, 500 mg po bid x 5 days Tetracycline 500 mg po qid x 5 days	Efficacy of treatment not established and should be reserved for patients with severe disease or immuno-suppression
Campylobacter jejuni	Erythromycin, 250-500 mg po qid x 7 days	Ciprofloxacin, 500 mg po bid x 7 days Doxycycline, 100 mg po bid x 7 days	May not alter course unless given early or for severe sx. Resistance to erythromycin has been described.
Chlamydia trachomatis	Tetracycline, 500 mg po qid x 7 days	Erythromycin, 500 mg po qid x 7 days	Prolonged course (3-4 wks) for LGV serovars.
Clostridium difficile	Vancomycin, 125 mg po q 6 h x 7-10 days Metronidazole, 500 mg po tid x 7-10 days	Bacitracin, 25,000 units po qid x 7 days Cholestyramine, 3 gm packet qid x 7-10 days	Vancomycin is preferred for severe disease. Discontinuation of implicated antibiotic is often adequate.
E. coli ETEC, EPEC, EIEC, EHEC, EAEC	Bismuth subsalicylate 60 ml qid x 5 days Sulfa-trimethoprim 1 DS po bid x 5 days	Trimethoprim, 200 mg po bid x 5 days Doxycycline, 100 mg po bid x 5 days Ciprofloxacin, 500 mg po bid x 5 days	Efficacy not established except for enterotoxin producing strains, eg ETEC (traveler's diarrhea).

Agent	Preferred	Alternative	Comment
Food poisoning Clostridium perfringens, Staph. aureus, Bacillus cereus, Listeria	None		Self-limited and toxin mediated: antimicrobial treatment is not indicated.
Plesiomonas shigelloides	Sulfa-trimethoprim, 1 DS po bid x 5 days	Tetracycline, 500 mg po qid x 5 days Ciprofloxacin, 500 mg po bid x 5 days	Experience with therapy is limited.
Salmonella typhi Typhoid fever	Chloramphenicol, 50-60 mg/kg/day in 4 doses po or IV until improved, then 30 mg/kg/day to complete 14 day course	Sulfa-trimethoprim, 160 mg trimethoprim as 1 DS po or IV bid x 14 days. Ampicillin, amoxicillin cefoperazone, and ceftriazone are other alternatives	Dexamethasone (3 mg/kg x 1, then 1 mg/kg q 6 h x 48 hr) for delerium, coma or shock.
Carrier	Ampicillin or amoxicillin 100 mg/kg/day + probenecid 500 mg po qid x 4-6 wks	Sulfa-trimethoprim	Cholecystectomy for gallstones.
Salmonella (other)	Sulfa-trimethoprim 1 DS po bid x 2 weeks Ampicillin, 2-6 gm po or IV/day x 3-14 days Amoxicillin, 2-4 gm po/day x 3-14 days	Ciprofloxacin 500 mg po qid x 3-14 days	Antibiotics should be restricted to patients with underlying debility or severe symptoms (enteric fever) AIDS patients may require long term suppressive treatment with ampicillin or ciprofloxacin

Agent	Preferred	Alternative	Comment
Shigella	Sulfa-trimethoprim 1 DS po bid x 5 days Ampicillin, 500 mg po or 1 gm IV qid x 5 days	Ciprofloxacin, 500 mg po bid x 5-7 days Nalidixic acid 1 gm po qid x 7 days	Ampicillin is preferred drug for sensitive strains. Ciprofloxacin preferred for strains resistant to ampicillin and TMP-SMZ.
Vibrio cholera	Tetracycline, 500 mg po qid x 2-3 days	Erythromycin, 500 mg po qid x 2-3 days Furazolidine, 100 mg po qid x 2-3 days	
Vibrio sp. (V. parahaemolyticus, V. fluvialis, V. mimicus, V. hollisae, V. furnissii, V. vulnificus)	Tetracycline (as above - see comments)		Efficacy of treatment is not established and should be reserved for severe disease.
Yersinia enterocolitica	Sulfa-trimethoprim 1 DS po bid x 7 days		Efficacy of treatment not established, especially when instituted late. Therapy with agents other than TMP-SMX has not been studied.

Agent	Preferred	Alternative	Comment
Parasites			
Cryptosporidia	Spiramycin, 1 gm po tid (investigational - see comments)		Efficacy of spiramycin is not established. Consider treatment only in chronic diarrhea in compromised host.
Balantidium coli	Tetracycline, 500 mg po qid x 10 days	Iodoquinol, 650 mg tid x 21 days	
Blastocystis hominis	(See comments)		Role as enteric pathogen is not clear. May treat with iodoquinol, 650 mg po tid
Entamoeba histolytica Acute dysentery	Metronidazole, 750 mg tid x 10 days then iodoquinol, 650 mg po tid x 21 days	Emetine, 1 mg/kg/day IM x 10 days then iodoquinol	Alternatives to iodoquinol as oral luminal-acting drug are: Diloxanide furoate, 500 mg po tid x 10 days; paromomycin, 500 mg po tid x 7 days Metronidazole may be given IV for severely ill patients (7.5 mg/kg q 6 h)
Mild disease	Metronidazole, 500 mg po tid x 10 days, then iodoquinol (as above)	Paromomycin, 500 mg po tid x 7 days Diloxanide furoate, 500 mg po tid x 10 days	

Agent	Preferred	Alternative	Comment
Cyst passer	Iodoquinol, 650 mg po tid x 21 days Diloxanide furoate, 500 mg po tid x 10 days Paromomycin, 500 mg po tid x 7 days	Metronidazole, 500-750 mg po tid x 10 days	Need to treat is arbitrary, but luminal amebicides are preferred
Giardia lamblia	Quinacrine, 100 mg po tid x 7 days	Metronidazole, 250 mg po tid x 7 days Furazolidone, 100 mg po qid x 7 days	Metronidazole is less effective than quinacrine, but better tolerated
Isospora belli	Sulfa-trimethoprim 2 DS po bid x 2 wks		Patients with AIDS and other immunosuppressive disorders usually require prolonged maintenance treatment
Viruses H. simplex	Acyclovir, 200 mg po 5x/day		Refers to treatment of herpes proctitis; recurrent disease may require maintenance with acyclovir, 200 mg po 2-5 x daily
Cytomegalovirus	Ganciclovir (DHPG, investigational), 5 mg/kg IV bid x 14-21 days		Efficacy in CMV colitis is not clearly established

B. Fecal Leukocyte Exam

Often present	Variable	Not present
Campylobacter jejuni	Salmonella	Vibrio cholera
Shigella	Yersinia	Enteroadherant
Enteroinvasive E. coli	Vibrio parahaemolyticus	E. coli
Exacerbations of	C. difficile	Enterotoxigenic
inflammatory bowel	Aeromonas	E. coli
disease	Plesiomonas	Food poisoning
	Enterohemorrhagic	S. aureus
	E. coli	B. cereus
		C. perfringens
		Viral gastroenteritis
		Adenovirus
		Rotavirus
		Norwalk agent
		Calicivirus
		Parasitic infection
		Giardia
		E. histolytica*
		Cryptosporidia
		Isospora
		Small bowel overgrowth
		"AIDS enteropathy"

* Frequency associated with blood.

URINARY TRACT INFECTIONS

I. Management recommendations (reproduced with permission from Kunin CM, Amer J Med 71:851.1981)

Group	Ease of Management	Type of Patient	Clinical Characteristics	Organism	Probability of Tissue Invasion	Therapy
I	Excellent	Female, child or adult	Few previous episodes; reliable, with good follow-up available; less than 2 days between onset of symptoms and treatment	Usually E. coli sensitive to most agents	Low	One dose amoxicillin, sulfonamide, TMP/SMZ, kanamycin
II	Good	Female, child or adult	Few previous episodes; follow-up poor	Usually E. coli sensitive to most agents	High or low	3–10 days Prophylaxis for closely spaced recurrences
III	Fair	Female, child or adult	Many previous episodes; history of early recurrence, or diabetic, or renal transplantation	Variable, tends to have more resistant bacteria, susceptibility tests essential	High	4–6 weeks Prophylaxis for closely spaced recurrences
IV	Fair	Male, adult	Recurrent infections, some underlying anatomic abnormality	Variable, susceptibility tests needed	High, often prostatic colonization	4–12 weeks Prophylaxis for closely spaced recurrences
V	Poor	Male or female	Neurogenic bladder, large volume residual urine	Variable, susceptibility tests needed	High	Intermittent catheterization (treatment for symptomatic infections only)
VI	Very poor	Male or female	Continuous drainage required	Variable, susceptibility tests needed	Very high	Indwelling catheter closed drainage (treatment for sepsis only)

Note: TMP/SMZ = trimethoprim with sulfamethoxazole.

II. Management recommendations of Medical Letter consultants (Medical Letter 23:69, 1981)

A. **Asymptomatic infection:** Treat only pregnant women and children.

B. **Single dose regimens:** Advocated for uncomplicated infections in non-pregnant females with dysuria-frequency syndrome who are likely to return for follow-up urine cultures in 48-72 hours.
   1. Amoxicillin (3 gm)
   2. Sulfisoxazole (2 gm)
   3. Trimethoprim (160 mg) - sulfamethoxazole (800 mg) (1 DS tab)

C. **Pyelonephritis:** Treat 10-14 days, usually with an aminoglycoside, betalactam or trimethoprim-sulfamethoxazole selected by in vitro sensitivity tests.

D. **Relapses:** Patients with recurrent infections involving the same bacterial strain according to speciation, serotyping and/or in vitro sensitivity tests should: **1)** be investigated for anatomical abnormality, calculus, prostatitis, etc; **2)** be treated two additional weeks if no abnormality is found.

E. **Prophylaxis**

   1. **Regimens: a)** Trimethoprim 40 mg - sulfamethoxazole 200 mg (½ tab) every other day.

      b) Nitrofurantoin, 50 mg daily (risk for serious reactions, especially pulmonary fibrosis)

      c) Infections clearly related to intercourse: may be prevented with single dose of an antimicrobial taken after intercourse.

   2. **Duration:** Usually 6 months; if symptoms recur frequently when prophylaxis is discontinued, it may be reinstituted for 2 years or more.

F. **Radiologic investigation:** Intravenous pyelogram is advocated for: **1)** Girls < 6 years; **2)** girls or women with recurrent infections; **3)** males regardless of age; **4)** pyelonephritis; **5)** Failure to respond to antibiotics

G. **Catheterized patient:** Treat only for symptomatic infections; antimicrobial prophylaxis has no established merit.

III Definitions of bacteriuric syndromes (Reprinted with permission from: Wilhelm MP and Edson RS, Mayo Clin Proc 62:1027,1987*

Syndrome	Definition
Lower urinary tract infection	Lower urinary tract symptoms† + urine culture with $\geq 10^5$ bacteria/ml
Acute cystitis	Lower urinary tract symptoms + urine culture with $\geq 10^5$ bacteria/ml
Acute urethral syndrome	Lower urinary tract symptoms + 10^2 to 10^5 bacteria/ml or venereally transmitted agent (for example, *Neisseria gonorrhoeae, Chlamydia trachomatis, Herpes simplex*) or no identifiable pathogen
Acute pyelonephritis	Upper urinary tract symptoms‡ + urine with $\geq 10^5$ bacteria/ml
Asymptomatic bacteriuria	No symptoms + urine culture with $\geq 10^5$ bacteria/ml
Recurrent bacteriuria	Recurrent lower urinary tract symptoms§ + urine culture with $\geq 10^2$ bacteria/ml
Relapse	Recurrent infection with same bacterial strain
Reinfection	Recurrent infection with different bacterial strain
Complicated bacteriuria	Urine culture with $\geq 10^5$ bacteria/ml with associated structural abnormality of the urinary tract§ (for example, involvement with stones or catheter)

* All syndromes usually associated with pyuria (≥ 8 leukocytes/mm^3 unspun urine).
†Dysuria, urgency, frequency; suprapubic pain.
‡Fever, rigors, flank pain, nausea, prostration.
§May be asymptomatic.

IV Outpatient management of urinary tract infections (Adapted from Wilhelm MP & Edson RS: Mayo Clin Proc 62:1025,1987)

Prophylaxis
Preferred
Trimethoprim-sulfamethoxazole, ½ tab q d or q o d
Macrodantin, 50 mg tabs, 1 tab q d
Trimethoprim, 100 mg tabs, ½ tab q d

Alternatives
Cephalexin, 250 mg tabs, 1 tab q d
Methenamine mandelate, 1 gm tabs, 1 tab q 6 h
Methenamine hippurate, 1 gm tabs, 1 tab q 12 h

Treatment
Trimethoprim-sulfamethoxazole 2 DS tabs
Amoxicillin, 500 mg caps, 6 caps (3 gm) } single dose
Sulfisoxazole, 500 mg tabs, 4 tabs (2 gm)
Trimethoprim-sulfamethoxazole, 1 DS tab q 12 h x 3 days or 7-10 days
Amoxicillin, 250 mg caps, 1 cap q 8 h x 7-10 days
Trimethoprim, 100 mg tabs, 1 tab q 12 h x 7-10 days
Nitrofurantoin macrocrystals, 100 mg caps, 1 cap q 6 h x 7-10 days
Nalidixic acid, 1 gm caps, 1 cap q 6 h x 7-10 days
Norfloxacin, 400 mg tabs, 1 tab q 12 h x 7-10 days
Tetracycline, 250 mg cap, 1 cap q 6 h x 7-10 days
Ciprofloxacin, 250 mg tab, 1 tab bid x 7-10 days

V. Cost of oral drugs commonly used for urinary tract infections

Antimicrobial agent and regimen	Wholesale price for 10 day supply*
Ampicillin: 500 mg po qid	$ 6.00** ($13.00)
Amoxicillin: 250 mg po tid	$ 5.00** ($6.30)
Amoxicillin + clavulanate (Augmentin): 250 mg po tid	$31.00
Carbenicillin (Geocillin): 380 mg po qid	$42.00
Cephradine (Anspor, Velosef): 250 mg po qid	$18.00** ($30.00)
Cephalexin (Keflex): 250 mg po qid	$14.00** ($30.00)
Ciprofloxacin (Cipro): 500 mg po bid	$37.00
Doxycycline (Vibramycin): 100 mg po bid	$ 4.00** ($41.00)
Methenamine mandelate: 1 gm po qid	$ 2.00
Methenamine hippurate (Hiprex): 1 gm po bid	$10.00
Nalidixic acid (NegGram): 1 gm caplet po qid	$31.00
Nitrofurantoin (Furadantin, Macrodantin): 50 mg cap po qid	$ 4.80
Norfloxacin (Noroxin): 400 mg po bid	$42.00
Sulfisoxazole (Gantrisin): 1 gm po qid	$ 4.40** ($10.40)
Tetracycline: 100 mg po qid	$ 2.40** ($5.20)
Trimethoprim: 100 mg po bid	$ 3.60
Trimethoprim-sulfamethoxazole (Bactrim,Septra): 1 DS po bid	$ 3.80*** ($12.80)

* Approximate wholesale prices according to "American Druggist Blue Book"
1988-1989 (Prices to patient will be higher).

**Price is provided for generic product if available; price in parentheses is for
representative brand product.

167

SEXUALLY TRANSMITTED DISEASES

CDC recommendations: adapted from MMWR 34 (Supplement) 75S-108S, 1985 and 36 (Supplement) 1S-18S, 1987

Organisms

I   Neisseria gonorrhoeae

Forms of resistance

Notation regarding antibiotic resistance of Neisseria gonorrhoeae that prompted 1987 CDC modifications of the 1985 treatment recommendations:

a. Penicillinase producing N. gonorrhoeae (PPNG): plasmid-mediated; escalating importance throughout the U.S., with 16,000 cases in 1986; accounts for a great majority of treatment failures.

b. Chromosomal resistance to penicillin (CMRNG): resistance is not due to betalactamase production; strains may be multiply resistant (tetracycline, cephalosporins, spectinomycin, other aminoglycosides) infrequently associated with treatment failures; prevalence not well established.

c. High level resistance to tetracycline (TRNG) which is not problematic with revised treatment recommendations that have eliminated tetracyclines as first line agents.

Surveillance: Primary aim is to detect PPNG

a. Non-endemic area: PPNG accounts for < 1% of strains.

b. Endemic area: PPNG accounts for 1-3% of strains.

c. Hyperendemic: PPNG accounts for > 3% of strains.

Management recommendations

a. Non-endemic area: Penicillins, ceftriaxone, or spectinomycin if penicillin or ampicillin are employed; routine susceptibility testing and test-of-cure are mandatory (ceftriaxone is a highly desirable alternative).

b. Endemic areas: Ceftriaxone (or spectinomycin) treatment preferred for selected public and private providers in neighborhoods with increased prevalence of resistant strains; antimicrobial sensitivity testing of strains from treatment failures, isolates from children and isolates from patients with complicated infections (disseminated GC infection, PID and ophthalmia).

c. Hyperendemic areas: Ceftriaxone (or spectinomycin) treatment preferred for all providers.

A. Treatment

1. Uncomplicated infections in adults: urethritis/cervicitis

   - Ceftriaxone, 250 mg IM combined with a tetracycline* (preferred)

   - Ampicillin, 3.5 gm po x 1 or amoxicillin, 3.0 gm po x 1, each combined with probenecid, 1 gm po and a tetracycline*

- Aqueous procaine penicillin G, 4.8 million units IM
  (2 sites) plus probenecid, 1 gm po and a tetracycline*

* Tetracycline, 500 mg po qid x 7 days or doxycycline, 100 mg po bid x 7 days
(the routine tetracycline regimen is for an anticipated concurrent chlamydial
infection). With contraindication (pregnancy or prepubertal children) or
intolerance: erythromycin base or stearate, 500 mg po qid x 7 days.

2. **Salpingitis:** See pelvic inflammatory disease

3. **Pregnancy:** Ceftriaxone (preferred), amoxicillin or ampicillin
    regimen as above, but with an erythromycin in place of
    tetracycline: erythromycin base, 500 mg or erythromycin
    ethylsuccinate, 800 mg po qid x 7 days; penicillin allergy, use
    spectinomycin, 2 gm IM combined with erythromycin.

4. **Gonococcal infection at other anatomical sites:**

    a) **Pharyngeal:** Ceftriaxone (preferred) or aqueous procaine
       penicillin regimens (as above, but without tetracycline for
       homosexual men).

    b) **Rectal in homosexual men:** Ceftriaxone (preferred) or aqueous
       procaine penicillin regimen (as above, but without tetracycline);
       for penicillin allergy use spectinomycin, 2 gm IM.

       Rectal infections in women: Use regimens listed for
       uncomplicated infections with tetracycline.

    c) **Disseminated gonococcal infection (DGI or arthritis-dermatitis
       syndrome):**

       - Ceftriaxone, 1 gm IV/day for 7 days* (preferred)
       - Aqueous penicillin G: 10 million units IV/day for at least 3
         days followed by amoxicillin or ampicillin, 500 mg po qid to
         complete at least 7 days total therapy*
       - Amoxicillin, 3.0 gm or ampicillin, 3.5 gm, each with
         probenecid, 1 gm followed by ampicillin or amoxicillin, 500
         mg po qid for at least 7 days total therapy*
       - Cefoxitin, 1 gm IV or cefotaxime, 500 mg IV qid for at least
         7 days*
       - Cefotaxime, 500 mg IV qid for at least 7 days*

    d) **Meningitis:** Third generation cephalosporin IV or high dose IV
       penicillin x 10-14 days.

* Combine with 7 day oral course of tetracycline, 500 mg po qid,
doxycycline, 100 mg po bid, erythromycin base, 500 mg po qid or
erythromycin ethylsuccinate, 800 mg po except for homosexual men.

e) **Endocarditis:** Third generation cephalosporin IV or high dose IV penicillin x 1 month.

f) **Ophthalmia (adults):** Hospitalize and treat with: Ceftriaxone, 1 gm IM or IV x 5 days; another effective third generation cephalosporin in equivalent doses (cefoxitin, 1 gm IV qid or cefotaxime, 500 mg IV) qid x 5 days or aqueous penicillin, 10 million units IV/day for 5 days.

5. Penicillin resistant strains: (See above notation)

a) **Penicillinase-producing N. gonorrhoeae (PPNG):**
Detect with test for betalactamase

- Ceftriaxone, 250 mg IM + tetracycline
- Spectinomycin, 2 gm IM + tetracycline

Pharyngeal infection: Ceftriaxone, 250 mg IM or Trimethoprim-sulfamethoxazole (720 mg/3600 mg), 9 tabs/day po in single dose x 5 days.

- Ceftriaxone, 250 mg IM
- Spectinomycin, 2 gm IM

b) **Chromosomally mediated resistant strains (CMRNG):**
Detect with agar dilution (preferred) or disc diffusion susceptibility test to determine sensitivity to penicillin, tetracycline, spectinomycin, cefoxitin and ceftriaxone.

6. Special considerations:

- Sexual partners: Women and heterosexual men exposed within the past 30 days should be seen, cultured and treated with a regimen for uncomplicated gonococcal and chlamydial infection

- Follow-up: Culture infected site 4-7 days after treatment completed, including rectal cultures for women

- Syphilis: Activity of ceftriaxone is not clearly defined so that patients with syphilis should be treated according to guidelines below

- Treatment failures: Ceftriaxone 250, mg IM or spectinomycin, 2 gm IM; all post treatment isolates of N. gonorrhoeae should be tested for antibiotic sensitivity

- Penicillin allergy: Cross reactivity with third generation cephalosporins is very rare; ceftriaxone should be withheld from only the occasional patient with an immediate or anaphylactic reaction to penicillin

II Syphilis

A. Treatment (adult, non-pregnant)

1. Early syphilis including primary, secondary or latent of less than 1 year duration.

   - Benzathine penicillin G, 2.4 million units IM x 1

   - Penicillin allergy: Tetracycline, 500 mg po qid x 15 days

   - Penicillin allery and tetracycline intolerance: Erythromycin 500 mg po qid x 15 days (this is acceptable only if penicillin allergy is confirmed and compliance plus follow-up serology is assured).

2. Syphilis over 1 year (except neurosyphilis) including latent syphilis, cardiovascular syphilis or late benign syphilis

   - Benzathine penicillin G, 2.4 million units q week x 3 successive weeks

   - Penicillin allergy: Efficacy for alternative regimens not established and CSF exam mandatory

     a. Tetracycline, 500 mg po qid x 30 days

     b. Penicillin allergy and tetracycline intolerance: Erythromycin, 500 mg po qid x 30 days (this is acceptable only if penicillin allergy is confirmed and compliance plus follow-up serology assured)

3. Neurosyphilis:

   - Aqueous penicillin G, 12-24 million units IV/day x 10 days, then benzathine penicillin G, 2.4 million units IM weekly x 3

   - Aqueous procaine penicillin G, 2.4 million units IM daily plus probenecid, 500 mg po qid x 10 days; then benzathine penicillin G, 2.4 million units IM weekly x 3

   - Benzathine penicillin G, 2.4 million units IM weekly x 3 doses

   - Penicillin allergy: Confirm allergy and "consult expert"

4. Pregnancy:

   - Penicillin regimens as noted above

   - Penicillin allergy: Erythromycin regimen (above). This is acceptable only if penicillin allergy is confirmed and compliance plus serologic follow-up assured; if not: hospitalize and "consult expert"

5. HIV infection (MMWR 37:600-602,607-608,1988)
- Early syphilis: Treat as recommended above under "early syphilis", although some authorities recommend CSF exam and/or treatment with regimen recommended for neurosyphilis.

- Syphilis > 1 yr: CSF exam and treat accordingly.

- Neurosyphilis (symptomatic or asymptomatic) and patients with syphilis > 1 yr who refuse CSF exam:
  (1) Aqueous penicillin G: 2-4 mil units IV q4h x 10 days.
  (2) Aqueous procaine penicillin G, 2.4 mil units IM/day + probenecid 500 mg po qid x 10 days.

B. CSF exam: Should be performed in patients with clinical symptoms or signs consistent with neurosyphilis. This exam is desirable for patients with syphilis of over 1 year duration.

C. Follow-up

Form	Follow-up quantitative nontreponemal test*	Expectation	Additional comments
Early syphilis	3,6 & 12 months post treatment	Nonreactive or low titer within 1 yr	CSF exam at last follow-up if alternatives to penicillin used
HIV infected	1,2,3 months and at 3 mo intervals		If titer does not decrease (2 dils) by 3 mo. for primary or by 6 mo. for secondary, or if titer increases (2 dils): re-evaluate for treatment failure versus reinfection, and examine CSF
Syphilis 1 yr	3,6,12 & 24 months post treatment	Titer declines more gradually	CSF exam as above
Neurosyphilis	Six month intervals at least 3 yrs. (see comments)		Clinical evaluation at 6 month intervals and repeat CSF exams for at least 3 years

* Nontreponemal tests = VDRL and RPR; treponemal tests = FTA-ABS, MHA-TP and HATTS

D. Indications for retreatment

1. Clinical signs or symptoms of syphilis persist or recur

2. Four-fold increase in titer with a nontreponemal test

3. A nontreponemal test showing a high titer initially fails to show four-fold decrease within one year

Retreatment: Recommended regimen is that advocated for syphilis over 1 year. Retreatment is advocated only once. A CSF exam is recommended before retreatment unless reinfection with early syphilis is established.

III Chlamydia trachomatis

A. Treatment (urethral, endocervical and rectal infection)

- Tetracycline, 500 mg po qid x 7 days

- Doxycycline, 100 mg po bid x 7 days

- Tetracycline contraindication: Erythromycin base or stearate, 500 mg po qid x 7 days or erythromycin ethylsuccinate, 800 mg po qid x 7 days

- Pregnancy: Treat as described for tetracycline contraindication with erythromycin. Women who cannot tolerate this regimen should receive half the suggested daily dose qid for at least 14 days

B. Sex partners: Examine for STD and treat using above regimen

C. Follow-up: Post treatment test-of-cure cultures may be omitted. If done and positive, retreat with one of the suggested regimens for the patient and any interim sexual partners

IV Genital herpes simplex

A. Treatment

1. First episode (genital or rectal infection)

   - Acyclovir, 200 mg po 5 times daily for 7-10 days initiated within 6 days of onset of lesions

   - Hospitalized patients: 5 mg/kg IV q8h for 5-7 days

2. Recurrent

   - Acyclovir, 200 mg po 5 times daily x 5 days if initiated within 2 days of onset

- Continuous (for patients with severe or frequent recurrences): 200 mg po 2-5 x/day for 18 months or possibly longer. This suppressive regimen is contraindicated in women who become pregnant during treatment

B. Sexual partners: Treatment not indicated

C. Pregnancy: Safety of acyclovir is not established

IV Chancroid (Hemophilus ducreyi) infection: Recommended treatment varies by susceptibility of strains in different geographic areas

- Ceftriaxone, 250 mg IM

- Erythromycin, 500 mg po qid x 7 days

- Alternative regimen: Trimethoprim-sulfamethoxazole, 1 double strength tablet (160/800 mg) po bid x at least 7 days

VI Lymphogranuloma venereum

A. Treatment (genital, inguinal and anorectal)

- Tetracycline, 500 mg po qid x at least 2 weeks

- Alternatives:
  Doxycycline, 100 mg po bid x at least 2 weeks
  Erythromycin, 500 mg po qid x at least 2 weeks
  Sulfamethoxazole, 1 gm bid x at least 2 weeks

B. Sex partners: Treat with a recommended regimen

C. Follow-up and management: Fluctuant nodes should be aspirated through uninvolved adjacent skin. Incision and drainage is contraindicated

VII Pediculosis pubis

A. Treatment

- Lidane (1%) lotion or cream applied to infested and adjacent hairy areas and thoroughly washed off after 8 hrs.

- Lidane (1%) shampoo applied 4 minutes and then thoroughly washed off. (Not recommended for pregnant or lactating women).

- Pyrethrins and piperonyl butoxide (non-prescription) applied to infested and adjacent hairy areas and washed off after 10 minutes.

B. Adjunctive: Retreat after 7 days if lice or eggs are detected at hair-skin junction. Clothes and bed linen of past 2 days should be washed and dried by machine (hot cycle each) or dry cleaned

C. Sex partners: Treat as above

VIII Scabies

A. Treatment

- Lidane (1%) 1 oz lotion or 30 gm cream applied to all areas of body below neck and washed thoroughly at 8 hr. (Not recommended for pregnant or lactating women.)

- Alternatives

  Crotamiton (10%) applied to body below neck nightly for 2 nights and washed thoroughly 24 hr after second application

  Sulfur (6%) in petrolatum applied to body below neck nightly x 3 nights. Patient may bathe before reapplying and should bathe 24 hrs after final application

IX Warts (Condylomata accuminata)

Location	Treatment	Comment
External genital and perianal	Cryotherapy, eg liquid nitrogen or CO_2 Podophyllin, 10% applied carefully to each wart and washed at 2-6 hr and reapplied weekly Trichloracetic acid (TCH) applied locally and repeated in 2-3 weeks Alternatives: Surgical removal, electrocautery, laser therapy	All treatments show high rate of recurrence Podophyllin is contra-indicated in pregnancy Women with external genital warts should have Pap smear
Vaginal and cervical		Usually detected by Pap smear or colposcopy with 3% acetic acid soak Treatment is complicated and requires consultant Podophyllin is not recommended
Urethral and meatal	Podophyllin as above for accessible meatal warts Alternative: Cryotherapy	Treatment requires consultant Urethroscopy required to detect intraurethral warts Podophyllin is not recommended for intra-urethral warts
Anal	Podophyllin or cryotherapy for warts accessible by anoscope Alternative: Electrocautery, cryotherapy or surgical excision	Some experts avoid podophyllin for anal warts Podophyllin is contraindicated

Syndromes - Female

I Pelvic inflammatory disease

A. Agents

1. Gonococcal PID: <u>N. gonorrhoeae</u>

2. Non-gonococcal PID: <u>Chlamydia trachomatis</u>, anaerobic bacteria + facultative gram-negative bacilli, <u>Actinomyces israelii</u>, <u>Mycoplasma hominis</u>

B. Indications for hospitalization: **1)** diagnosis uncertain, **2)** surgical emergencies cannot be excluded (such as appendicitis or ectopic pregnancy), **3)** pelvic abscess suspected, **4)** severe illness prevents outpatient management, **5)** pregnancy, **6)** patient unable to follow or tolerate outpatient treatment, **7)** failure to respond to outpatient treatment, **8)** clinical follow-up at 48-72 hours not possible.

C. Treatment

1. Antibiotics: <u>Outpatient regimen</u>

   Initial dose: Ceftriaxone, 250 mg IM x 1 dose.

   Followed by: Doxycycline, 100 mg po bid for 10-14 days.

2. Antibiotics: <u>Inpatient regimen</u>

Initial*	Oral follow-up**
<u>Preferred when GC or Chlamydia is suspected</u>	
- Doxycycline, 100 mg IV bid	Doxycycline, 100 mg po bid
+ cefoxitin, 2.0 gm IV qid	
<u>Preferred when anaerobes or normal flora is suspected</u>	
- Clindamycin, 600 mg IV qid	Clindamycin, 450 mg po qid
+ gentamicin, 2.0 mg/kg IV,	
then 1.5 mg/kg tid	

* Parenteral treatment to continue at least 4 days and 48 hrs after patient becomes febrile.

**Oral regimen to be continued to complete 10-14 days of treatment

3. Male sex partners: Examine and treat with regimen for uncomplicated gonococcal and chlamydial infection.

4. Follow-up: Outpatients should be re-evaluated within 72 hrs and patients not responding should be hospitalized. Test-of-cure cultures for organism isolated should be done 4-7 days after therapy is complete.

5. Intra-uterine device: Removal is recommended soon after antimicrobial treatment is started.

176

II Mucopurulent cervicitis

A. Diagnosis: **(1)** Mucopurulent endocervical exudate that may appear yellow or green on white cotton tipped swab (positive swab test); **(2)** gram stained smear of endocervical secretions shows over 10 PMN/oil immersion field or **(3)** cervicitis documented by cervical friability (bleeding when the first swab is taken) and/or erythema or edema within a zone of cervical ectopy.

B. Treatment

1. Gonococcal: N. gonorrhoeae found on gram stain or culture - treat for uncomplicated gonococcal infection (pg 168,169)

2. Non-gonococcal: N. gonorrhoeae not found on gram stain or culture - treat for C. trachomatis (pg 173)

III Vaginitis/vaginosis

A. Trichomoniasis

1. Usual treatment:
   - Metronidazole, 2 gm po as single dose
     Alternative: Metronidazole, 250 mg po tid x 7 days

2. Asymptomatic women: Treat as above

3. Pregnant women: Metronidazole is contraindicated in first trimester and should be avoided throughout pregnancy. Alternative is clotrimazole, 100 mg intravaginally hs x 7 days

4. Lactating women: Treat with 2 gm dose of metronidazole and suspend breast feeding x 24 hrs

5. Sex partners: Treat with 2 gm dose of metronidazole

6. Treatment failures: Retreat with same regimen. Persistent failures: Consider 2 gm dose daily x 3

B. Bacterial vaginosis (non-specific vaginitis)

1. Diagnosis: Non-irritating, malodorous, thin, white vaginal discharge with pH over 4.5, elaboration of fishy odor after 10% KOH, microscopic exam showing sparse lactobacilli and numerous coccobacillary forms in epithelial cells ("clue cells"). Cultures for Gardnerella vaginalis are not recommended.

Syndromes - Male

I <u>Urethritis</u>

A. Categories

1. Gonococcal

2. Non-gonococcal: Usually caused by <u>C. trachomatis</u> (40-50%) or <u>Ureoplasma urealyticum</u>

B. Diagnosis: Gram stain and culture of urethral discharge or urethral swab obtained with calcium amalgamate swab

1. Gram negative intracellular diplococci or positive culture for <u>N. gonorrhoeae</u>: treat for uncomplicated gonococcal infection (pg 168,169)

2. Gram stain shows > 5 PMN/low power field plus no intracellular gram-negative intracellular diplococci: Treat for <u>Chlamydia trachomatis</u> (pg 173)

3. Stain shows < 5 PMN: Patient should return for repeat test next morning prior to voiding

C. Persistent or recurrent NGU: Consider

1. Failure to treat sexual partner

2. Alternative causes of discharge

2. Sex partner: Treat only for Candida balanitis

- Nystatin, 100,000 unit tab intravaginally qd x 2 weeks

- Clotrimazole, 500 mg intravaginally x 1

- Miconazole nitrate or clotrimazole, 200 mg intravaginally qd x 3 days

- Miconazole nitrate or clotrimazole, 100 mg intravaginally qd x 7 days (cream and tablets considered equally effective)

1. Treatment

C. Vulvovaginal candidiasis (not considered an STD)

3. Sex partners: Treatment not indicated

- Alternative: Ampicillin or amoxicillin, 500 mg po qid x 7 days

- Metronidazole, 500 mg po bid x 7 days

2. Treatment

II Epididymo-orchitis

A. <u>STD form</u>: Usually occurs in young adults in association with urethritis without urinary tract infection or underlying GU pathology

Usual agents: <u>C. trachomatis</u> and/or <u>N. gonorrhoeae</u>

1. Treatment: Use regimens for uncomplicated <u>N. gonorrhoeae</u> infection

2. Adjuncts: Bed rest and scrotal elevation recommended until fever and local inflammation have resolved

3. Follow-up: Failure to improve within 3 days requires re-evaluation and consideration for hospitalization

B. <u>Non-STD form</u> (usually older men in association with GU pathology and/or UTI verified by positive urine gram-stain and culture)

1. Agents: Coliforms and pseudomonads (usual agents of urinary tract infections)

2. Treatment: Based on severity of disease and urine culture results

3. Adjunctive treatment as above

179

181